FIRST, DO NO HARM

FIRST
DO NO
HARM

Wrestling with the
New Medicine's
Life & Death
Dilemmas

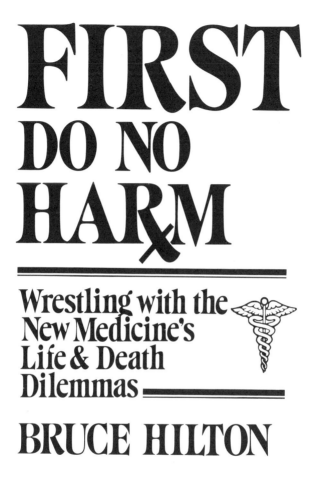

BRUCE HILTON

ABINGDON   PRESS

Nashville

FIRST, DO NO HARM

This book is printed on recycled, acid-free paper.

Library of Congress Cataloging-in-Publication Data

Hilton, Bruce.
    First, do no harm : wrestling with the new medicine's life and death dilemmas / Bruce Hilton.
        p.   cm.
    Includes bibliographical references.
    ISBN 0-687-13050-6 (alk. paper)
    1. Medical ethics. 2. Patients—Legal status, laws, etc. 3. Euthanasia. I. Title
R724.H53   1991
174′.2—dc20   90-42190
                                                                      CIP

MANUFACTURED IN THE UNITED STATES OF AMERICA

To Vern and Mary Hilton,
my first and best ethics teachers,
and an example for thousands more
in sixty years in ministry together

ACKNOWLEDGMENTS

*A*lthough they're in no way to blame for any deficiencies, this book owes a lot to others, especially these:

The Reverend Virginia Young Hilton, M.A., M. Div., R.N., life's companion, pastor, health-care professional, whose help in understanding the mysteries of medicine is only one of her many gifts to me over the years.

Martin Janis, M.D., partner in leading ten years of monthly Bioethics Grand Rounds at Brookside Hospital, and the doctors, nurses, and other professionals who taught me so much in the smoke and fire of those discussions.

David Hilton, M.D., for vision beyond the urgencies of the here and now.

Joanne Derbort, insightful editor of my columns in the *San Francisco Examiner,* from which many of these discussions were adapted, and Peter Bhatia, for the vision to suggest and run the column in a daily newspaper.

Clay Berling, Rick Schlosser, and Earle Atkinson, who wrestled with these issues over coffee on many mornings.

Bob Veatch, Bob Neville, and Marc Lappe, colleagues at the Hastings Center in the early 1970s, who generously shared information, insight, and encouragement when this was all new to me.

CONTENTS

INTRODUCTION
THE KING WHO DIED ON DEADLINE

Doctors have many secrets to keep, but few so awesome as the one Lord Dawson took with him to the grave. He had killed King George V, ruler of the British empire. Not by mistake. Not with a drug's unexpected side effects. He did it on purpose, by injecting his unconscious patient with three-quarters of a gram of morphine and one gram of cocaine. He did it because he thought a lingering death would compromise the king's dignity, and it was time for him to die.

Lord Dawson's act stayed secret for more than fifty years, finally becoming public in 1988 when his biographer revealed the notes the physician had made that night of January 20, 1936.

The seventy-one-year-old king had been seriously ill for only four days, but it was clear that he was dying, and that he could linger unconscious for a long time. Late in the evening, the Archbishop of Canterbury had prayed at the bedside. When he left, Dawson was alone with the king.

He had been told by the queen and by their son, the Prince of Wales, that they didn't want the king's life needlessly prolonged. About 11:00 P.M., after a while in thought, Dawson carefully filled two syringes and injected the fatal substances.

Then he called home and asked his wife to advise the prestigious *Times* of London to hold up publication of the next morning's edition. By midnight, the king was dead. The prince (who would abdicate within a year to marry an American divorcee) was now king. Dawson notified the *Times,* which rushed to press with a bulletin: "Death of the King: A peaceful ending at midnight."

Then Dawson wrote the details in his notebook, including this paragraph: "It was evident that the last stage might endure for many hours, unknown to the patient but little comporting with the dignity and the serenity which he so richly merited and which demanded a brief final scene."

He added a second rationale: He had hastened the king's death because he wanted the announcement to be "in the morning papers rather than the less appropriate evening journals."

And the *Times* of London got the scoop.

■　■　■

This is a book about life-and-death decisions, a book made necessary because so much has changed since Lord Dawson's day—and so much has remained the same.

For one thing, doctors have much less freedom to make secret decisions; their power is no longer unquestioned. The responsibility for ethical decisions in medicine has been handed over to you, the patient. Dawson had to wrestle with what it meant to follow the ancient code of doctors, "First, do no harm." Doctors still do, but now you share the burden—and the challenge.

Our society, and even our religious training, hasn't given us much help in facing the moral questions raised by the new medicine. But with a little advance thought and reading, your decisions can be as good as anybody's.

This book should help. It's a collection of snapshots, brief flashes at many problems from different points of view. Whether you read it straight through or open the pages to whatever segment catches your eye, I hope it intrigues and stimulates you to find out more.

It should start more arguments than it settles, because you're the decision-maker. I hope it will provoke you to thought and study, and, sometimes, to strong disagreement. Most of all, I hope it gives you a chance to think, ahead of time, about two kinds of events unavoidable in any life these days: The times when you'll have to wrestle with questions of life and death for yourself or somebody you love. And the times when health law and public policy are being made—a job too important to leave just to the lawyers, doctors, bioethicists, and other professionals.

Sacramento, California
April 15, 1990

PART ONE
GETTING ACQUAINTED
WITH BIOETHICS

---

*I*t's been more than twenty years since Carl Salamansky offered to buy somebody's kidney, but the moral issues he raised are still around to trouble us.

A reporter spotted Salamansky's classified ad in a New Jersey newspaper:

"Need kidney transplant. Will pay $3,000 to donor of suitable kidney. Intend to commit suicide if none found."

The reporter called the phone number given, and talked to a man in his late thirties who seemed thoughtful and rational.

"Yes, it's for real," Salamansky said. "My kidneys have failed. For a year, I've been going in twice a week for hemodialysis, having my blood filtered for six hours.

"I'm not doing well, and I've been on the waiting list for a transplant for eight months. But there just aren't enough available.

"So I placed the ad. If I can't get a kidney within a month, I don't want to go on living this way. I'll just end it all."

As it turned out, he got the kidney he needed (free) from a teenager killed in an accident—but then died from complications of the operation.

The questions raised by his case are typical of those considered in bioethics—the moral, social, and legal implications of advances in medicine and biology.

They are the unexpected side effects of the new medicine.

Salamansky's bold offer, at a time when transplants were still new and risky, forced people to begin asking questions such as:

• Is it ethically acceptable to try to buy part of someone else's body?

• Is it ethically acceptable to sell part of one's body? Is the occupant of the body its true owner? Or are we caretakers on behalf of the Creator—or Mother Earth, society, or some other power beyond ourselves? Since Salamansky's death many states have written new laws to forbid giving up an organ for profit, and to forbid a donor from designating the recipient. But enforcing such a law isn't always easy, and there still are too few kidneys for transplant.

• Does a person have a right to quit receiving a medical treatment that is keeping him or her alive? And is it suicide to do so? In recent years, new laws and court decisions have backed up the nearly absolute right of a patient to refuse treatment, even if it means death. And the courts have been clear that this isn't suicide. But there are exceptions. Utah courts, for example, stopped a thirty-five-year-old father from taking himself off a kidney machine, saying his responsibility to his two children outweighed his right to refuse medical treatment.

• Should a relative be allowed to donate? Often the person most likely to be a good tissue match for a transplant is a member of the family. But many physicians believe the pressure to donate, the fear associated with the donor operation, and the guilt if one doesn't really want to do it are so great that nobody should be confronted with such a choice.

• Which of the 50,000 people dying of kidney failure each year should get one of the rare available kidneys? Computer networks and a national policy make the decision less haphazard than it was in Salamansky's day, but there still are far too few donor organs to go around. And why is that?

• Many states have a donor card you can affix to the back of your driver's license if you want to make organs available. But some people say that's not enough. These people argue that the law should assume that all organs of fatal accident victims, for example, are available for transplant unless they carry a card stating otherwise. Would you agree?

• Should expensive procedures like transplants go only to those, like Salamansky, who can pay for them? If not, then who should pay? Believing that wealth isn't a good way to choose who gets to stay alive, Congress voted that Medicare should pay for life-saving dialysis and transplants for everybody who needed them. But that raised a new dilemma: Why not also hemophilia, the inherited "bleeders' disease," which can cost as much as $80,000 a year per person to treat? Or Alzheimer's, or any other chronic, expensive disease?

• A related question: Why spend something like $1 billion a year helping people whose kidneys have failed, and only a tiny fraction of that on research to prevent kidney failure? What if we had done the same thing with polio, spending all the money on iron lungs and almost none on a vaccine?

These are a few of the questions raised by just one skirmish in the medical revolution. Now take a quick look at a variety of other issues, getting a feel for the questions and how some people go about finding an answer.

Through the Ethical Maze to a Decision

A mother and her grown son stand by a hospital bed, surrounded by the privacy curtains and the hush of the intensive care unit. The man in the bed lies on his back, tubes in his nose and both arms. He seems to stare at the ceiling, but his eyes never move.

The mother says to her son, "The doctor wants us to decide. There's no chance Dad will wake up again, but he could live like this for months, maybe even years, as long as they keep feeding him through that tube.

"The doctor says she'll remove the tube if we give permission."

■ ■ ■

How would you go about finding an answer to that question? How would you arrive at a reasoned, appropriate decision?

Most of us don't know. Most high schools don't teach the discipline called ethics. Even in church school we tend to get a laundry list of do's and don'ts, rather than experience in making moral choices ourselves. The scriptures are silent on most of the dilemmas raised by the new medicine; there's hardly been time for experience and tradition to develop; reason is not much help amid the pain, fear, grief, strange machinery, and intimidating surroundings of a hospital.

So when we're faced with a tough ethics decision, we fall back on one of these three:

• We go with our "gut" feelings—ranging in degree of certainty from "I have a good feeling about this" to "I know I'm right."

• We look to the majority. We ask what "most people" would do. Or we poll the others around the bedside.

• We trust our conscience. Unlike feelings, conscience implies some tests—some thought and insight about events around us.

These factors are a start. But by themselves, they're little more than conditioned reflexes. Feelings can vary widely from hour to hour; the majority is often wrong, and conscience, while important, is too much a reflection of our conditioning to be reliable on its own.

There's no umpire, no societal "commissioner of baseball" to help us judge the ethical quality of an act or to hand down a ruling. But that doesn't mean there are no guidelines at all.

There are, in fact, three areas in which there is a good bit of agreement, and which we can use to begin analyzing the decision facing us:

Obligations. We don't act in a vacuum; our significant acts take place in relationship to others. A given act may be right or wrong, depending on whether it meets an obligation or violates it. The most obvious obligation is a legal contract. But there are many others, often unspoken: obligations of friendship, of family, of a profession, of citizenship, of trust, and of promises to keep.

Mother and son have an obligation to "take care of" Dad. What does that mean in the intensive care unit? Did he ever say what he would want in a situation like this? The doctor has an obligation to try to heal—but that may conflict with another obligation: not to extend suffering.

Ideals. These basic beliefs underlie the way we and our society act, although it doesn't always show. There's general agreement on ideals like justice, respect for persons, loyalty, telling the truth, caring about others.

How do wife and son reconcile the ideal of the sanctity of Dad's life with the ideal of quality of life? The doctor's concern for the well-being of relatives might lead to violation of a conflicting ideal, such as telling the truth.

Consequences. What will happen if we take the proposed action? Will it do more good than harm? Will it help more people than it hurts? What would happen if everybody in this situation made the same decision?

Ethicists differ about how much emphasis to give this factor. Will the family always feel guilty if they allow the feeding tube to be removed? What will be the impact of Dad's death? On him (will he be better off)? On others? What will be the impact on society if the act of withdrawing a feeding tube becomes an accepted practice?

■ ■ ■

In helping families make their own health-care decisions, I tend to emphasize ideals and obligations, turning to consequences as a "tie-breaker" when two of the ideals conflict. But whatever the balance, considering these factors along with what your feelings and conscience tell you will help you move toward a responsible decision.

Tough One for the Ethics Committee

Suppose you are a member of a hospital's Ethics Committee, one of the many lay people on such committees, and you've been called together to discuss the case below.

(This is a real situation, whose participants gave permission to describe it here.)

L is fifty-nine years old, a retired department-store buyer. She's in the hospital because a persistent pain in her right thigh turned out to be bone cancer.

A cancer specialist and a cancer surgeon have consulted with her family doctor, and they agree her best chance for survival is to amputate the leg as high as possible, right at the pelvis.

Without the operation, the cancer is likely to spread, and then L will not live very long. But the location means that an artificial limb will be difficult to fit, and that L will probably always be dependent on a wheelchair.

She has been distraught since she got the diagnosis. Her moods have swung between long bouts of crying, days of silent depression, and times of near-manic cheerfulness during which she denies that a problem exists.

J, her husband, has little faith in Western medicine and is dead set against the operation.

He wants to take his wife to an alternative-medicine clinic in west Texas, where health foods, various herbs, and body manipulation will be used to fight the bone cancer.

At one of the office visits, he told the surgeon, "The only thing you doctors can think of is to cut."

The daughters attend the Ethics Committee meeting and tell you they disagree with their father.

"It's Mother's only chance," says the older daughter, a homemaker and mother of two children. "I want my kids to know their grandmother and have her around as long as possible."

The younger daughter, an assistant professor of math, agrees. "How can we risk her life with some far-out theories, when there's a chance of keeping her alive? There are worse things than not being able to walk."

It has been hard to find out what L herself wants. Sometimes she has told the doctor and the family that she is ready to face the surgery and wants to have it. Sometimes she has cried that she "would rather be dead than to be so deformed and so dependent on everybody."

Since the desires of a competent patient are among the first things an ethics committee considers, a psychiatrist has been asked to evaluate L's distraught state. Is she able to make a decision for herself?

The psychiatrist reports that L often seems rational and lucid, but often doesn't, and concludes, "I cannot confirm her mental competence." The committee has gathered at noon, bringing lunch on trays from the cafeteria to the board room. Not everybody could come on short notice, but two doctors and a nurse are there, along with a lawyer who practices in the community, an ethicist who teaches philosophy at a community college, and you.

"Well, here's the case," the committee chair says, "and as I told you over the phone, it's not an easy one."

You shuffle through the papers—the summary; the reports of the primary physician, the consultants, and the psychiatrist; photocopies of pages from a lawbook and from an ethics text.

"As you know," the chair says, "it's not our job to make a decision for L. Our job is to make sure all the options are spelled out for her—or, if she's not competent, for her family and doctors. But as we work through the possibilities, we're certainly going to learn what one another's opinions are."

As she talks, your mind plays back the questions you feel are crucial, the ones the committee kept coming back to in the year of monthly training sessions:

Who should be the decision-maker in this case? What is strictly medical in this case, for the doctors to decide, and what are the non-medical factors for L or her surrogates to decide? What are the choices? How does L feel about values like autonomy, professional responsibility, the sanctity of life, mobility, and independence? Did she ever discuss situations like this?

You also find yourself asking, "Does she believe in life after death? And should that make a difference?"

And, inevitably, crowding in from the back of your mind, "What would I do if it were me? Or my mom?"

Values Behind Your Choices

The bioethics decisions required of us by the new technology in medicine won't go away, and won't get any easier to make.

Many of them are true dilemmas—decisions for which no answer is really acceptable. But each time, somebody has to come up with an answer. As a sign on a wall says, ''Not to decide is to decide.'' It's not as oppressive as it sounds. Making such a decision for ourselves, after hearing all those who have advice to give, is an affirmation of free will, of responsibility, and of our uniqueness as individuals.

A little practice helps, of course.

To get some experience at being your own bioethicist, consider this series of decisions—choices being made by tens of thousands of couples every year. Imagine that you're half of such a couple, sitting in a doctor's office, hearing the results of amniocentesis, a test early in pregnancy.

The doctor has just told you that the baby-to-be has a birth defect or an inherited disease—one of those described below—and that there is no cure for such a condition. The terrible choice, he tells you, is either to end the pregnancy—not an easy thing for anybody—or carry the child to term and live with the results. (Imagine, for the purposes of this exercise, that you can accept abortion in some situations, and that there is a prenatal test for each condition described here.)

The question is this: Which, if any, of these conditions would make you decide not to have the baby?

Case 1. The child will die within a few days of birth, no matter what measures are taken to save it (e.g., anencephaly).

Case 2. The child will grow normally for about six months and then retrogress, eventually becoming blind, deaf, and paralyzed, dying at about a year of age (e.g., Tay-Sachs disease).

Case 3. The child can expect to live as long as nineteen years, perhaps more, of a relatively normal life—except for time-consuming lung exercises and expensive medical treatments every day (e.g., cystic fibrosis).

Case 4. There will be normal life until about forty, and then ten to fifteen years of mental and physical deterioration, eventually fatal (e.g., Huntington's disease).

Case 5. Normal life expectancy, but with severe mental retardation, requiring lifelong guardianship at home or in an institution (e.g., some Down syndrome).

Case 6. Normal life expectancy, retarded but capable of learning and eventually getting a job in a sheltered workshop (e.g., some Down syndrome).

Case 7. Normal life expectancy, average intelligence or above, but paralyzed from the neck down (e.g., some spina bifida).

Case 8. Normal life expectancy, average intelligence or above, but paralyzed from the waist down (e.g., some spina bifida).

■　■　■

After you've guessed what your choices would be (none of us knows for sure unless we're actually in the situation), go back and consider why you chose the way you did. What values of yours show up in the choices you made? For example, length of life, amount of suffering, quality of life, and sanctity of life.

Or the idea of "normal." What does it mean? Who defines it for you? Ethics decisions often require balancing two opposing values—a fetus' "right" to be born, for example, against his or her "right" to an abundant life, to "quality" of life. And is the expected quality of life of the parents and other children in the family a factor or not?

Did you think of the effect on society if your decision were a common one? Or on generations a hundred years from now?

A Crystal Ball: Would You Use It?

If you could look far into the future and see how you were going to die, would you want to know?

That question used to be hypothetical, the kind of thing you kick around at a late-night college bull session. And then the new medicine came up with an early childhood test that tells, forty years in advance, whether you're going to have Huntington's disease (HD).

HD is inherited, and it's a bad way to die. You deteriorate neurologically, over ten to fifteen years. You gradually lose control of body movements, while showing symptoms of mental illness. For most people, it strikes in the late thirties or early forties. Before it hits, there is no warning.

When it first appears, victims often are accused by their families of being secret drinkers. Their speech is slurred, their walk unsteady, their temper often violent and unpredictable. Marjorie Guthrie says that when her folk-singer husband, Woody, first showed the symptoms, she noticed him walking down a New York street, leaning as if he had his guitar slung over his shoulder. But there was no guitar.

HD is inherited through a dominant gene, which means that if either of your parents had the disease, you have a fifty-fifty chance of having it too. But until a few years ago, you had no idea beforehand whether you were going to be a winner or a loser in the Russian roulette of genetics. If your parents told you about the risk when you were a child, you had decades of uncertainty ahead. Should you train for a career, marry, have a family, plan for retirement?

But like so many other discoveries in the new biology, a new test changed the ethics questions. The question had been, "How shall I handle the fact that I have a 50 percent chance of getting the disease?" Now it was, "Do I really want to know?" and could be, "How shall I live my life, knowing it will end early and amid much suffering?"

The unlucky half could know for sure, as early as someone wanted to tell them, that they would die of HD. The odds would be 100 percent. The only room for hope would be in the sudden discovery of a cure—only a faint possibility in the near future, since an inherited disease is rooted in the genetic map that's in every cell of the body.

What would this sudden surety do to the person who tests positive? Much of the bizarre behavior of the last forty years has been blamed on awareness that nuclear death lurked nearby. Would the life of a young man or woman with HD—but no symptoms yet—be an intensified version of that nuclear-age mind set?

Or would denial, one of our most powerful mental processes, take over, convincing the person that he or she is in the lucky half of those at risk? This seemed to be the most common approach when a research center in Boston began offering the tests. Of all the people at risk, only two hundred and fifty inquired about the tests. Of those, only forty-seven actually came in to be tested. And of those, nineteen withdrew before they could learn the results.

Which brings us down to the hard questions:

If you were a parent of small children at risk, what would be the right thing to do? Test, or not? Tell, or not? At what age would you decide? Might the knowledge of what lay ahead make you overindulgent or overprotective? Has the child a right to know? A right not to know? How does one make such a decision for another?

Would you be willing to tell all your blood relatives of the result, risking the stigma and superstition surrounding inherited disease in order that they might know they were possibly affected?

Would you advise your affected children not to have children of their own? Would you agree with the suggestion from some geneticists that your kids should be forbidden by law to have children?

For most of us, these questions are theoretical, even though our answers reveal our most deeply felt attitudes about life, risk, death, and what it means to be human. But for the spouses, children, relatives, and friends of those at risk for HD, the new breakthrough is all too real—a "Twilight Zone" crystal ball.

Cures for Which There's No Disease

So, having small breasts is a disease. Worse than that, it is a deformity.

That's the official opinion given by the American Society of Plastic and Reconstructive Surgeons, when it asked the Food and Drug Administration to ease restrictions on breast implants. The argument went like this:

"There is a body of medical information that these deformities [small breasts] are really a disease which, in most patients, results in feelings of inadequacy, lack of self-confidence, distortion of body image, and a total lack of well-being."

Something is sick here, all right, but is it the woman with the "deformity"? Or a society that makes her feel inadequate?

Here we are in a national medical crisis, unable to care for maybe one-fourth of the people in the country, with babies and old folks dying for lack of medical help. And there are physicians out there eagerly inventing new diseases. You can't load all the blame on the surgeons, of course. They're just the fixers in a society with a distorted idea of what makes a human being valuable. And questions of what is disease, and who defines it, involve a whole lot more than just the one specialty.

Psychiatrists face the hard question, "What is illness?" all the time, because a broken psyche doesn't show up on an X ray like a broken bone.

For a while in the 1970s, they were treating "abnormal aggression" by using a charged silver wire to create a scar in the brain. It was a while before somebody pointed out that 80 percent of the people being treated this way were women. It didn't take too long to figure out why: The same behavior our society saw as abnormal aggression in a woman was rewarded as get-up-and-go in a man.

For a while the psychiatrists defined homosexuality as a disease, mainly because nobody challenged homophobia in the society at large in those days. Then at a convention they voted to take it off the list of diseases. It was a conclusion that made sense, but the way it was reached, by political process, was less than satisfactory.

And now, with the new medical technology, redefining disease may be a growth industry. Shortness, for example. Until genetic engineering made human growth hormone available, we just accepted the idea that people come in different sizes. Now, if you want offspring everybody will look up to, find a doctor willing to inject HGH, and thereby overcome the formerly incurable "disease" of short stature.

Prenatal diagnosis makes it possible to find out whether a fetus is male or female and to abort the unwanted sex—a rare event but enough to cause biologist Dr. Estelle Ramey to ask, in this sexist society: "Is being born female now a genetic disease?"

But it's the cosmetic surgeons who raise the most questions about redefining sickness. Many of their patients are people disfigured by accidents, burns, or birth defects, and a skilled, caring surgeon can make their lives better. But what to do with the increasing number who are victims of society's preoccupation with an "ideal" body?

One answer would be to use the prestige of physicians to change public attitudes that measure a woman's worth by the shape of her body.

"Because It's the Right Thing to Do"

Quaker Oats did what Socrates, Kant, and Thomas Aquinas never got around to doing. They made ethics a registered trademark. Remember their TV and magazine ads, a while back, featuring the kindly but direct gaze of Wilford Brimley? A popular character actor, he looked like everybody's grandfather—the one who has seen it all, wrestled through all the confusing issues of life, and now, in the calmness of advanced age, knows the answers. He was just the man for selling breakfast cereal. No fancy words about minimum daily requirements or cholesterol. It took him just one phrase to tell you why you should buy the product:

"Because it's the right thing to do."

Trademarked. In the magazines there's a little "TM" next to the last letter, telling us that Quaker has exclusive rights to the phrase. For selling cereal, at least.

A TV character who gives off similar vibrations, in a show likely to be in reruns well into the twenty-first century, is Angela Lansbury of "Murder, She Wrote." The show is not really about murder, but about a person of integrity and common sense, staying true to herself while surrounded by the sleaziest and greediest collection of amoral characters the writers can invent.

The reason for bringing all this up is not to give the actors or the oat people a hard time, but to consider the phenomenon—to wonder out loud about the powerful attraction these fictional personae have.

Here are several theories, each ripe for some Ph.D. candidate in psychology, ethics, or nutrition to turn into a dissertation:

• Maybe things are so confused these days, we're hungry for somebody to make moral decisions for us—to flat-out tell us what to do. Cults get their power because of this, relieving believers of the responsibility for choosing. What comfort there is in surety!

• Maybe we've had to turn to fiction because there aren't enough models of integrity in real life. In a simpler age we looked to public figures as models of rectitude—or, closer to home, the parson or the schoolteacher. Truth-in-packaging has revealed that every walk of life can be a journey on feet of clay—probably a good development, but one with its down side.

• Or maybe the phrase, *what's right* has lost its meaning altogether, and has a place only in fiction, as nostalgia. It's possible that there are whole generations of Americans who do a thing because it works. Because it pays off. Because it gives us an advantage. Because it feels good. Because everybody else is doing it. Because it's hip. Because it's not hip. Because somebody tells us to. Because somebody tells us not to. Because a commercial convinced us to. But rarely because "it's the right thing to do."

Meanwhile, the questions get harder, not easier. In the intensive care unit, in the genetic engineering lab, at the toxic waste dump, at the arms talks, in the health-care planning committee the need is as great for thoughtful people of integrity as it ever was.

It isn't enough to have only the cereals enriched with—excuse the pun—moral fiber.

Potholes in the Yellow Brick Road

What do you do when your myths don't work any more?

No, not Zeus or Persephone. I mean the myths we've lived by most of our lives. A myth, as Joseph Campbell reminded us so vividly in many appearances on public TV, is a story that helps us make sense out of our world. It may be factual or not; it is "true" for those who live by it. In Sam Kean's words, it's "an invisible stew of unquestioned assumptions" that shape the way we look at things and, thus, how we act. Our own personal and societal myths are usually invisible to us, but we all have them.

We chuckle at the bushman who prays to a river, but are just as much influenced by a myth—Mother Earth as inexhaustible provider—in our reluctance to recycle cans or save water.

Matters of sickness and health are no different. Powerful myths have shaped the way we feel about getting sick and how we try to get well. And if our health-care system is in a mess, it's probably because the world has changed while our myths haven't.

A few examples:

• **Disease as the Wicked Witch.** When the Salk and Sabin vaccines were discovered in the 1950s, they put a swift end to the dreaded disease polio. It was like the moment in the *Wizard of Oz* when Dorothy splashed water on the Wicked Witch—who immediately melted down to nothing because water was the one thing that could kill her.

For most of this century, we've thought of health care that way: as the search for a specific antidote to each disease. There must be a pill or an injection for every illness, and if we haven't discovered one yet, we will.

That was the myth that moved us when the government declared war on cancer in the 1970s, pouring millions into a search for a cure. But we had already run out of diseases that could be dispatched so easily; cancer is not one of them. Like most of the remaining threats to health, it resists treatment and may be caused not by an identifiable bug but by genetics, the environment, or even by the fact that we inevitably get older.

In a day when emergency rooms are flooded with victims of assault-rifle shootings, drug abuse, AIDS, and the strokes and heart attacks of an increasingly older population, the "magic bullet" myth doesn't work.

• **The body as Tin Woodsman.** In the age of transplants, we've come to see our bodies as machines, as collections of replaceable parts. "If I only had a heart," the Tin Woodsman sang. And we snap in a plastic heart, or plug in a breathing system, hoping to keep the machine running, maybe indefinitely.

But the body is an organism, not a machine, and its parts are inextricably interrelated. There's a limit to the substituting you can do, or how long you can artificially delay the last natural act of living: dying.

• **The doctor as Wizard.** Since most of us believe subconsciously that death is a curable disease, we demand that someone find the cure, and the doctor is our choice for the job.

Some doctors relish the role of Wizard, but an increasing number are glad to be relieved of it. Unreal expectations have led to a public backlash, bringing to mind Dorothy's cry, "You're a bad man!" and the Wizard's gentle response: "No, I'm a very good man. I'm just a very bad Wizard."

• **The patient as Munchkin.** Just as the passive Munchkins looked to Dorothy to free them from the Witch, we lay people see ourselves as relatively helpless in matters of health. We feel dependent upon the power and expertise of others to rescue us. But the focus is changing, from expert-centered to people-centered. We're taking responsibility for decisions that affect our health, including diet and exercise.

Meanwhile, around the world, health care systems are improving fastest where small groups of lay people have met to ask: What is it about our health that concerns us most? And what can we do about it? Expertise is still valuable, but it is much more effective within priorities the people have set for themselves. Myths are a way of understanding the world around us. As you consider the dilemmas in the rest of the book, maybe you can come up with some myths that do work for health care today.

A Step for Humans—or onto the Slope?

Remember the first time you stood at the top of the playground slide—the high one—and tried to make yourself take that first step onto the slippery surface?

If so, you may be able to appreciate the concern of people who believe that some exciting research from Sweden and England puts us all at the top of a fast and dangerous slope.

"The slippery slope" is a phrase that turns up often in ethics arguments, used by those who are afraid that an unprecedented and apparently beneficial act will open the door to similar, less acceptable acts.

This scary vision happened with the announcement that brain cells from an aborted fetus were implanted into two Britons suffering from Parkinson's disease. A doctor told the press that both patients had been sent home, so much better that they were able to stop the medicine they'd been taking before the operation.

Their recovery was dramatic: One of the pair had the transplant just two weeks earlier.

The implanted tissue seems to stimulate the body to produce dopamine, a brain chemical lacking in people with Parkinson's. It relieves the jerky, uncontrollable movements and the gradual loss of muscle control.

The operation is simple. With only a local anesthetic, a small hole is drilled in the skull and the tiny bits of tissue are slid between folds of the brain. Tissue from a fetus is used because its immune system has not developed enough before death to cause the usual transplant rejection in the recipient.

There are medical questions—how long the effects will last, for example—but the procedure has amazing promise for people sentenced to a hellish existence.

Why, then, are some people so worried? Why, in April 1990, did the U.S. Department of Health and Human Services turn down a request by government researchers to try the brain implant, using aborted fetuses?

Some, of course, are those whose single issue is protection of the fetus at all costs. Most of the rest consider the brain implant for Parkinson's a worthwhile and moral procedure, but are afraid it's the top of a downhill slide. They point to the woman who has declared she'll get pregnant and abort the fetus so its brain cells can be available to her father, who is severely disabled with Parkinson's disease.

The pressure for the wondrous substance will be so great, some say, that hospitals will end up selling aborted fetuses, either legally or on a black market. Since one in four pregnancies ends in a spontaneous abortion—a miscarriage—there would be plenty of material available.

If the laws stop that, they say, the next step could be women who get pregnant for the purpose of producing fetal tissue donors. By then the fetus, rather than a potential human worthy of respect, would have become in society's eyes a commodity—a therapeutic device, even though produced in a human container rather than in a factory vat.

And how would you stop this? With legislation forbidding abortions for relatives of Parkinson's sufferers? With legislation against all abortions, thus reversing the hard-won right of women to have a choice?

Some members of this debate, however, say the slippery slope is not the relevant issue. No new development is risk-free, they say; the risk of misuse is not a strong enough argument to halt work with great potential for good. The real issue here, they say, is the choice between competing rights and needs: those of a dead fetus and those of a person crippled by Parkinson's disease. For me, that would not be such a hard choice. The opportunity to free a living, thinking, suffering man or woman from a torturing disease is clearly the greater good.

Meanwhile, we must work on such questions as: How can we safeguard the dignity of the fetal cadaver? Can we find such efficient ways to gather tissue from spontaneous abortions that we don't need to look to other sources? That may keep us off the slippery slope; if not, it may be a risk worth taking.

PART TWO
BODY PARTS: DONORS AND DILEMMAS

---

*I*t didn't look like much of a Christmas for Dubby and Diana Wilcox of Bald Knob, Arkansas. Their three young boys had been killed a month earlier in a fire that gutted the Wilcox home. To add to their grief, a nurse had asked them whether they would donate the boys' organs to be transplanted. The Wilcoxes said no. But they spent a little time thinking about what the boys might have wanted, and finally gave permission.

The gift meant that a fourteen-year-old boy from Pennsylvania and a thirty-three-year-old woman from North Carolina received life-saving liver transplants. Four Arkansas residents got new kidneys. And forty-eight-year-old Mary Wilson of Jacksonville, Arkansas, received a new heart, from ten-year-old Jared Wilcox. She celebrated Christmas at home with her family—a Christmas she hadn't been sure she would live to see.

And another thing happened. The Arkansas regional organ recovery agency said it had received ''more organ donor referrals in November than in any month in our history.'' It said the reason probably was the Wilcoxes' widely publicized decision, in a Christmastime that might otherwise have been unrelieved misery, to give the gift of life.

Transplanted into a Political Storm

When Christiaan N. Barnard made the first incision for the first successful heart transplant, he had thought through many of the medical problems. But how could he have forseen, more than two decades ago, the human and political fallout we see today?

For example, the Israeli who needed a new heart, lying in a bed just five miles from the dying young Palestinian with a transplantable heart? As the *Los Angeles Times* reported it, twenty-year-old Mohammed Nasser had been one of seven young men fatally shot by Israeli troops while carrying the outlawed Palestinian flag in a funeral procession. Israeli TV told of the shootings and reported that Nasser and another victim were in an Arab hospital, dying but on life support.

In Jerusalem, a wealthy Jewish man heard the broadcast. Yehuda Israel pricked up his ears because his brother, Yehiel, was in a Jerusalem hospital with a failing heart. A transplant was the only hope. Through important friends who knew prominent Arabs, he made inquiries about the dying young men. He passed the word that he would pay a large sum of money to surviving relatives for a transplantable heart.

But for Hassan Nasser, brother of the dying Mohammed, there were two problems. Moslems consider it wrong to give away an organ of a living person—and believe a person is alive as long as the heart is beating. Artificial support was keeping Mohammed's heart beating. The second problem was political and geographical, and went back a thousand years: "They kill us, and then they ask for such a thing," Hassan said. "I rejected it right away."

Some older Arabs pled for the donation, as a gesture of peace toward the Israelis, but the younger family members were firmly against it.

In Jerusalem, Yehiel Israel underwent a heart-valve operation that failed, and died three days later.

In the occupied territory, Mohammed Nasser was buried secretly.

On second thought, Barnard might have had a clue, a faint warning, of such events. One of his first transplants, in racist

South Africa, put the heart of a black man into the body of a white. He was not prepared for the storm of protest over this "race-mixing." But he couldn't have forseen the dying teenaged boy in California who willed his heart to the high school girl he had loved, but who hadn't loved him. The heart saved her life. Nor could he have known that hospitals would become competitors for donor hearts, often refusing to make known the existence of a donor even when they didn't have a recipient, hoping that one would turn up. Research grants, journal articles, promotions, and prizes were at stake. That situation continued until 1988, when new federal regulations required reporting of all potential donor hearts, and allocation by an independent agency.

Who could have foreseen the hope and joy brought by transplants on babies under six months old—twenty-three of them at one California hospital alone? The youngest, operated on when she was only three hours old, was at home and well thirteen months later.

And, sadly, who could have known that sometimes professional ambition would overrule the welfare of these tiny patients, as in the case of the baby taken home by her mother to die of a congenital heart defect. The surgeon-researcher went to the home and persuaded the mother to bring the baby back—to receive a baboon heart. The extra life she got could be measured in days.

Could Barnard have foreseen that bereaved families would find such solace in permitting a donation? Or that all transplants would someday have to be tested for HIV, the AIDS virus?

Maybe it's the mythical role of the heart as center of our being that has involved it in so many bioethics issues. Or our belief that medicine someday will stave off death permanently. Whatever it is, it's obvious that when we consider the heart transplant, we look at it not with our minds, but with our hearts.

Everybody Was Asking
the Wrong Questions

In covering the heart-wrenching story of six-year-old Alex Vlahos's struggle against leukemia, reporters had plenty of questions. But Alex's case raises troubling questions—questions of ethics—that nobody got around to asking. You may remember Alex, whose parents' search for a bone-marrow transplant flashed briefly on the nation's picture tubes in the summer of 1989.

Who could resist? A six-year-old's courageous struggle, a last chance to live, the desperate search for a matching donor, and even the heroic sports figure—Giants pitcher Dave Dravecky, himself a cancer victim—lending encouragement and raising money.

The publicity brought in more than $200,000 in donations, to pay for the expensive testing of would-be donors and for the procedure itself. He received the marrow in September, three months after the story first broke. Six months later, in March 1990, Alex gave in at last to the leukemia.

But the questions won't go away. For example, the questions of media ethics: To what extent should the news media let themselves be used for advocacy publicity, even in the most sympathetic of causes? Once the pattern is set, does justice call for all the thousands of leukemia victims' cases to be similarly publicized? And, with reporters swarming all over the Vlahos's front yard, how should we balance the family's right to privacy when it conflicts with the public's right to know? And where is the fine line between reporting news and manufacturing it?

Reporters agonize over the first two questions much more than most readers and viewers realize. And most don't worry about shedding their professional objectivity in a case like this one. They wanted Alex to get the bone marrow transplant that might cure his leukemia, and were willing to help all they could.

But some news agencies were drawn into a nasty side of the story. And not just drawn in. They ended up helping create it. Susan Vlahos, Alex's mother, was regional marketing director for a cosmetics firm. She knew how to communicate to a wide audience, and Alex's need was soon known nationwide.

But after a month-long search for a donor, she began criticizing the agencies conducting the search. In the days before instant news, there would have been time to evaluate her weary remark. Was it really news? Was it the most important thing she said? Maybe so, maybe not. But there apparently was no time for evaluation. The criticisms were on videotape.

TV assignment desks reacted, the automatic responses clicked in, and camera crews were on their way. On their way where? Well to interview the searchers, of course, and ask them to respond to Susan Vlahos's charges. The news media did this because that's the way it's done, not because there was any need or reason to.

Without ill intent—and equally without serious thought—they created a story that needlessly hurt the Vlahos family. It hurt the people trying to help them, and it hurt the news media too. And the real story got lost in the kind of controversial confusion that TV feeds on.

A second and more important question: Nobody ever asked why the search for publicity and money for Alex was necessary. Nobody pointed out the utter lack of sense in the way we deal with a problem like Alex's.

In most of the world's developed nations, Alex Vlahos would simply have gone to a hospital where his medical needs would have been met out of the taxes his family and others paid. Not in this country. Here we hardly question the idea that life-saving health care should be available only to those somehow able to raise the cash. The real question: By what strange logic have we come to accept as normal the specter of Alex's parents on TV, pleading for nickels and dimes to save their son's life?

Liberty and Transplants for All

Ironically, one of the most important transplant stories of the '80s hardly made the inside pages. It was about a big change in the way we decide who gets them. Since the first transplant, and especially since the use of cyclosporin A to avoid rejection, the toughest problems about transplants have not been medical, but moral: Who got the life-saving organs when there weren't enough to go around? Who decided? And on what basis?

In a land of "justice for all," the job of getting healthy organs together with worthy candidates in an equitable way was much tougher than you might think. Among the glitches:

• **Lack of organs.** There are enough kidneys for only 20 percent of the people who need them. And 20 to 40 percent of the heart-transplant patients die while awaiting a donor heart.

• **Lack of communication.** An information system to connect organs and donors across the country was slow in coming, partly because of administration foot-dragging in spending money appropriated for it by Congress.

• **Competition.** As transplant agencies have multiplied, accusations of organ-grabbing, publicity-grabbing, and grant-grabbing—all related—have grown and sometimes have surfaced in the press. A doctor's research papers must be about his or her own work; letting somebody across the country do the transplant won't help you get a chairmanship or a grant renewal.

• **Public appeals.** When Phil Donahue's show brought together a little girl and a liver, the world went "awwww"—

except for other couples whose children had been waiting longer and resented line-crashing. President Reagan's appeals on behalf of half a dozen children helped draw attention to the overall problem, but also created a serious injustice for the hundreds of dying children who didn't have such help.

• **Money.** Although the scandal was papered over, it is clear that a number of scarce kidneys on the East Coast were going into the bodies of Saudi Arabian princes and others able to pay well above the going rate.

• **The good news.** The government and the transplant surgeons finally got together in a historic Chicago conference and decided that distribution of organs was going to be more just. The 100 organ-procurement agencies, the 200 transplant centers, and all the tissue-typing labs were going to have to work through the United Network for Organ Sharing (UNOS). Either that, or lose Medicare, the major source of transplant money.

UNOS, established a few months before the conference by the medical profession as an information-sharing computer network, keeps a list of approximately 10,000 people who are waiting for organ transplants—including 9,000 for kidneys, 300 for hearts, and 300 for livers. Now the other shoe was dropping: UNOS became the central place to be notified of all organs available for transplant.

UNOS allocates the kidneys to people who are the best match, and who rank highest on a point system. Among the items giving the most points are how long they've been on the waiting list, how urgent the need is, and how near they are to the available organ.

The long-overdue system is leading to better-matched kidneys for more patients, a higher rate of success for transplants, and millions of dollars saved in dialysis (kidney machine) costs.

45

More important, it introduced the idea of justice into one small part of the United States health care system.

Giving When It Doesn't Hurt Any More

Sometimes the wonders of modern medicine make things worse instead of better. When, for example, the doctor says to you, "We could save her life with a transplant, if we could only find a donor. But we've checked the network, and there just isn't one available." All the miracles of the new organ-matching computer system, of microsurgery, of anti-rejection drugs, and post-operation care don't do you a bit of good if there's no donor in the picture. It would be easier to take if transplants had never been made possible.

So the next step in solving the moral issues of transplants came as a government regulation. Whenever a patient dies in a hospital that gets Medicare or Medicaid payments, the family must be asked whether they are willing to allow organs or tissue to be donated.

Soon after the regulation came out, I found myself in a breakfast meeting at a hospital where I'm the ethics consultant. We were there to plan how the hospital would put the new regulations into practice. One thing was made clear from the start: The question was to be asked only "when appropriate," and there was to be no pressure on the family to say yes. But the question was to be asked.

Seems like a simple regulation, and more sensible than most federal rules. But the discussion was far-ranging, raising many issues. Here's a behind-the-scenes glimpse at some of the implications:

• Who would ask the question? There were no physicians at

the meeting, although some had been invited. But it had already been agreed that, in this hospital, nurses would be the ones to approach the family. The rationale was that nurses spend more time with the family and know the family better than the doctor usually does. But there was another reason. Doctors—usually protective of their turf—were glad to turn this over to the nurses because they didn't want the job. Dealing with the death of a patient is already too difficult for many doctors. At the meeting, one doctor was quoted: "I can't believe this is a law. You'll have to show it to me. The AMA would never allow such a law."

• **Paper work.** People from medical records and the medical staff office wanted to know if a special team would come in to remove the donated organ. (Yes.) Then what arrangements could be made—at 3:00 A.M., for example—to grant staff privileges to the visiting surgeons?

• **Technicality.** If a patient is declared dead one day but remains in the hospital on artificial support two more days, until the donor operation, what is the date of discharge? (Medicare and Medicaid are pretty picky about these things; the "discharge" date is when the patient dies.)

• **Payment.** After the death, who pays for the special nursing care, special medicines, and then the donor operation? (The new unified federal transplant program.)

• **What donations to accept.** While hearts and kidneys get all the publicity, bone and other tissue is also needed, as well as corneas, lungs, pancreases, and livers.

• **Family reaction.** Would families be angry at being approached at such a time? The visiting expert told us, "More families are offended by not being informed of the chance to give. Most families see it as a way to let the one they love live on."

• **Families and donor cards.** Even if a patient carries the donor card on the back of his or her driver's license—a legal document—no hospital will take the tissue or organs without family consent, because they don't want trouble.

• **Giving your all.** Wouldn't it be simpler just to give one's whole body? Probably not. Organ and tissue donation can be done without visible scarring—important to many families. Besides, in the state where we were meeting, donating organs is free. But to give your body away, you must pay $100.

The Forgotten Hero on the Table

There's a forgotten hero in many of the news stories about kidney transplants. And the ethical questions involving this person make other transplant problems—tissue-matching, long-distance races against time, organ rejection—seem simple. The forgotten hero is the relative who donates a kidney, and who is the patient's best chance for long-term survival.

New anti-rejection drugs have made transplants from dead donors more successful than ever, but the live relative is still the best donor. And yet, for ethical reasons, a few transplant teams won't let relatives be donors. Before we get into the ethics of it, consider what's happening backstage, while the spotlight is on the patient whose life is being saved:

The donor is undergoing a serious operation. It will last anywhere from four to six hours, and leave a scar from the navel around to the backbone—"ruling out bikinis forever," one donor told an interviewer.

A twenty-two-year-old single mother, she described the process to a medical-magazine reporter: Her two-and-a-half-year-old nephew had been on kidney dialysis and fed by plastic tube since birth. When his condition began to get worse, doctors began cross-matching the family for possible donors. Only two aunts were a medical match, and one of those declined because of health problems and concern for her family.

The other aunt had a three-year-old daughter, but said, ''It's hard to see a little kid suffer when you know you can help him.'' She decided to go ahead.

She was tested for pregnancy and for the AIDS-causing HIV virus. Her heart and kidneys were checked, and the cross-match was repeated. After each test the doctors asked whether she wanted to change her mind. ''If I chose to back out, they would save face for me by telling the boy's parents the test results weren't acceptable.'' Then she was counseled in turn by the boy's doctor, a nurse, a psychiatrist, and a group of other would-be donors. Twice the whole family met with the transplant team, and each time she was given a chance to change her mind.

She checked into the hospital the day after the little boy did. There was one last cross-match, X rays, insertion of IV tubes in each arm, and sleep. She woke up in the recovery room, nauseous and vomiting. On the second day she was allowed to see the youngster, who was feeling much better than she was. And after a week she was able to go home.

The transplant center in St. Louis had been sensitive to the key ethics questions:

• Were potential donors given every opportunity to decline, without implied guilt?

• Did the donor understand not only the risk and the life changes required, but the uncertainty involved in all medical procedures?

• How could the team respect the would-be donor's right to perform an altruistic act, while being sure there's no coercion by social or family pressure, fear of what people will say, guilt, a death wish, or any other unspoken pressure?

The difficulty of these questions is the reason some doctors just tell would-be living-relative donors they don't cross-match, avoiding the whole thing, and why others at least reserve the right to refuse the offer.

Three months after going through all this, the donor told a writer that she still received counseling, trying to deal with "a hesitation to get on with life" and with a diet that restricts spicy foods, coffee, and alcohol.

"I worry that someday I might have to go on dialysis, and although my doctors say this is far from likely, I remember seeing [my nephew] on the machine and I worry." But don't get her wrong. She has no regrets.

PART THREE
THE NEW RESEARCH: NOISY ISSUES FROM QUIET LABS

———————————

*I*s it ever right to use scientific data that were gathered in a morally unacceptable way? Specifically, should data from the Nazi doctors' horrendous experiments during the Holocaust be added to the pool of information going into a research project today—a project that might help save lives? It's a classic bioethics dilemma, and it popped up again because the chief of the Environmental Protection Agency said no to that question.

Lee M. Thomas, administrator of the EPA, said he had deleted from an agency report data that the Nazis got from phosgene-gas experiments, which they performed on prisoners in World War II concentration camps.

Low doses of phosgene are used to make pesticides and plastics, and the EPA was concerned about its effect on users. The purpose of the study was to spell out what various doses of the gas would do to human beings. The first draft of the study pointed out that in 1943 and 1944, fifty-two prisoners were exposed to phosgene by Nazi doctors, to see how much it took to kill them. The purpose of the experiment was to find an antidote to the gas in case it was used as a weapon—as it had been in World War I.

The inclusion of the Nazis' data set off a debate among scientists at the EPA, and eventually triggered a letter to Thomas from a group of those scientists who were opposed. At first glance, the arguments seem plain enough.

One side argued that the abysmally immoral way the information was gathered rules out its use; no end is great enough to justify this means. The others believed that data are neutral, and that no matter how regrettable the means of their collection, they were now in the pool of knowledge that can be used toward something good.

It isn't quite that clear, though, is it? Some people will argue, for example, that the pool of modern scientific data is already polluted—that maybe even the preponderance came from research aimed at killing people, in the wars—hot and cold—that have preoccupied research since 1939.

Other people will argue that you can no more rule out the results of the Nazis' immersion of helpless prisoners in ice water (to see how long it took them to die, and thus design ditching gear for pilots) than you can rule out computers, whose first major use was building the atomic bomb.

The medical literature is full of data on the effects of radiation on humans, gathered among the survivors of the Hiroshima and Nagasaki atomic explosions. Do the growing questions about the morality of those bombing missions also raise questions about the propriety of using the radiation data?

In these cases, some would deplore the means by which the information was gathered, but argue that now that we have the information, it should be put to good use. They might even argue that this would be a way of salvaging something good from the evil done to the prisoners and bomb victims.

One could point out other examples of data gathered in ethically unacceptable ways, if not quite as monstrous as the Nazis'. For example, would you rule out the work of Dr. Robert Gallo, this country's leading researcher on the AIDS virus, because it is widely believed that he appropriated the crucial virus samples and data from France's Pasteur Institute?

My own reaction—one man's opinion—is this:

• We must try to make sure that in gathering data, we never again come close to the Nazis' ghastly dehumanizing practices—and this includes all experiments on humans without their full, informed consent.

• We must be vigilant against any argument that theft, deceit, or cutting corners in research is justified ''for the greater good.'' We should be prepared to expose professionals who live by such a code.

• And no, I would not use the Nazi data. Even the suggestion that we might we willing to profit in any way from that heinous crime is repugnant—and could give the impression that, in a pinch, we might abandon our scruples to get crucial data. We don't need any piece of information that badly.

This Time We're the Guinea Pigs

We can work up a fine head of steam over the outrageous medical experiments the Nazis performed on the Jews, gays, and rebels in the concentration camps. But where's the outrage over our own experiments on helpless subjects?

When the Nazi doctors wanted to know how long a downed aviator could survive in the ocean in winter, they just put a few gay and Jewish prisoners in a freezing tub. The justification was this: They needed the information, and this was the only way to get it. The research subjects' welfare and wishes were irrelevant. After World War II, the Nuremberg Code was designed to stop that kind of logic, but it didn't. Consider these three timely cases:

Experiment Number One: U.S. Army release of bacteria into the air—170 times in nine years at the Dugway Proving Ground, seventy miles from Salt Lake City. They're the same bacteria that caused one death and much sickness when the Army turned them loose over San Francisco one time.

These germ-warfare experiments violate the Nuremberg

Code's first provision: "The voluntary consent of the human subject is absolutely essential." But retired Major General William Creasy, former head of the program, says the public can't be told when they're being sprayed with infectious agents because they would panic. He justified the Dugway experiment this way: Germ warfare agents "are designed to work against people, and you have to test them in the kind of place where people live and work."

That kind of logic—strangely familiar—will keep the program going. Dr. Leonard Cole of Rutgers wrote in the *New York Times:* "Army officials steadfastly assert their right to test outdoors anywhere in the country, including in urban areas. The Pentagon insists—despite a pile of contrary evidence—that the tests are harmless."

Experiment Number Two: Exposing students to a highly toxic insecticide. The state of California was under pressure to ban Zolone, because during the previous autumn it had made seventy-eight farmworkers sick, thirteen of them ending up in the hospital.

The president of the Tulare County Farm Bureau—a paid consultant to Zolone's manufacturer—arranged an experiment to test its safety. He rounded up forty "volunteers" who would enter the grape fields fourteen days after spraying with Zolone. (The state Health Services Department recommends a thirty-five-day wait.) They would do this each day for six days, and then have their blood and urine tested.

He found his volunteers at the job placement office of Porterville Community College, where "students might need extra money." The $100 a day he offered also seemed to quiet any qualms the out-of-work students had about cancer or genetic defects.

Were they, as the Nuremberg Code demands, "able to

exercise free power of choice, without the intervention of any element of force, fraud, deceit, duress, over-reaching, or other ulterior form of constraint or coercion''?

Experiment Number Three: A five-organ transplant on a three-year-old girl. Little Rolandrea Dodge got a new liver, pancreas, stomach, small intestine and part of a large intestine, in what Pittsburgh Children's Hospital called a life-saving—and experimental—procedure.

Even though we all want this little tyke to survive the fatal disease she was born with, and as much as we'd like to coat her struggle with sentimental sugar, we need to be honest: Rolandrea was a research subject, not a patient. The agony she went through gave her only a few more weeks of life.

Strapped there, trying to understand, do you suppose she meets the part of the Nuremberg Code that says research subjects should have ''sufficient knowledge and comprehension of the elements of the subject matter . . . to make an understanding and enlightened decision''?

Why Frostban Gets People So Heated Up

The night before, vandals had trampled the strawberry patch. Now, in the morning, company officials greeted the press with a show of confidence, wearing ''Frostbuster'' T-shirts and bringing their kids to play just outside the fence.

Environmentalists had filed one last suit, but the four-year battle was over. Company scientists sprayed a genetically altered substance called Frostban on the strawberries. They were finally able to test their data and breathe a sigh of relief.

To reporters, the scientists showed a hurt but not angry face. Like Charlie Brown, they asked, ''Why is everybody always pickin' on me?'' Their own answer to the fuss over releasing gene-split experimental substances in the air was to blame an ignorant public, roused to paranoia by kooks and eco-fanatics. But this approach was no more honest or useful in resolving the dispute than was the trashing of the strawberry patch by somebody on the other side. The fact is that there were also responsible, knowledgeable scientists raising practical and ethical questions about the frost-killer bacteria.

The questions included concerns about a ''runaway bug,'' and about researchers evaluating the safety of procedures in which they also have a big stake. But those issues could be dealt with.

The toughest question, I think, was the one raised repeatedly by Dr. Robert Sinsheimer, former chair of biology at Caltech and chancellor of the University of California-Santa Cruz. It has to do with the evolutionary consequences of DNA research—bridging eons of natural selection. From bacteria to beetles to Nobel Prize-winners, all us living things evolve in an environment that shapes us. When a life form is removed from the control exerted by its natural environment, the results are unpredictable.

An example: Homesick British immigrants brought a few rabbits to Australia in the late nineteenth century, to make the landscape more familiar. Free of the natural predators among whom they had evolved in England, those rabbits bred into a horde and ate their way through millions of acres of farms, many of which are still wasteland, 100 years later. Australia had to build the longest fence in the world, 5,000 miles from coast to coast, to hold back the rabbits. Australian farmers still lose crops to the ravenous rabbits. There are many other examples, including Florida's walking catfish and the irrepressible eucalyptus brought from Australia to California by a Methodist missionary.

But bringing a gene from one life form into another is much

more basic. Sinsheimer says we're short-circuiting a billion years of evolution with the very stuff of life. It could be either harmless or disastrous. Sinsheimer spells out the dilemma of the concerned science watcher: "Somehow it is presumed that we know, a priori, that none of these clones will be harmful to man or to our animals or to our crops or to other microbes—on which we unthinkingly rely. I don't know that and, worse, I don't know how anyone else does."

Meanwhile in the strawberry patch, scientists were hoping a new life form, created by DNA transfer, would replace natural bacteria that live on the surface of the fruit. Frost forms on a protein produced by the natural bacteria. But the manufactured bacteria don't have the gene to make that protein. If the researchers are right, it would mean cheaper, healthier fruit for all of us. Frost destroys something like $1.6 billion worth of U.S. crops every year.

But who worries about the alternatives? Certainly not the company that paid for the research, which hopes for $300 million a year in sales from Frostban—and which had been fined just a year earlier for an illegal and unannounced release of altered bacteria into the air of downtown Oakland, California. Probably not the government, whose regulatory teeth have been pulled by DNA industry lobbying.

One who does worry is Dr. David Pimentel, who says present controls aren't enough. He wants OSHA and the EPA firmly in charge. He wants fuller testing in labs and greenhouses and then on remote islands before U.S. farmers' fields are exposed. And he wants inspection by teams that include ecologists, wildlife specialists, and public-health professionals.

Pimentel, no kook, has chaired the Board on Environmental Studies for the National Academy of Sciences. Professor of insect ecology and agricultural sciences at Cornell, he has been a consultant on this subject to the National Institutes of Health, the Environmental Protection Agency, and the congressional Office of Science and Technology. He says, "Although there is only a small chance that such an organism could cause an environmental problem, a single mistake could lead to a major disaster."

That's why many people wanted a more cautious approach to the strawberry patch. And why the public, remembering Australia's rabbits, should never be afraid to ask the scientists, "What's up, Doc?"

Research Nobody Wants to Do

Scientists down through the centuries have called it a sin, a sickness, or a crime. It involves at least one person in every ten. And yet twenty-four centuries after Plato made one of the first clumsy attempts to explain homosexuality, we don't have much more scientific data on it than he did. In fact, it's hard to find any subject about which science seems so determined to remain ignorant.

There was a spurt of interest in the nineteenth century. Moreau spoke of hereditary "taint"; followers of Darwin decided homosexuality was a reversal of evolution; Freudians were the first to raise seriously the idea of cure. But there were no controlled scientific studies.

In the 1970s psychologists and psychiatrists decided that it is not sickness that makes some men and women most attracted to others of their own sex. Most scientists gave mental—if not emotional—assent to the idea that this was not a sin, a sickness, or a crime.

A consensus grew that there is no one cause of same-sex attraction; both constitutional and developmental factors are likely. Beyond that, as Dr. Vern Bullough says, science is right where it was fifty years ago: "There seem to be far too many variables involved to offer any simple answer."

But Bullough, who compiled a major bibliography, said of the 4,000 medical titles on homosexuality since 1870, "The majority offer no new insights, and most can be dismissed as pseudoscience."

It doesn't take a genius to see why the vacuum exists in research. Data are hard to get because society imposes a life of secrecy on most of the subjects. Research grants are few because there's little or no political pressure to fund such work.

Just as important: Scientists reflect society's homophobia. They're afraid to show interest, for fear of being thought gay. This should be no surprise. The existence of homosexuality makes many people deeply uncomfortable. It threatens some basic notions: It deviates from the "norm"—reason enough, in most eyes, for suspicion. It doesn't result in more children for society. It violates the social roles prescribed for each sex. In some situations, it raises the gut fears of male-dominated society by penetration of the male body.

Basically, though, society is homophobic out of ignorance. It is a closed loop: Bigotry forces most lesbians and gay men to remain closeted; this leaves a knowledge vacuum to be filled by more bigotry. The cost of this ignorance is high, and it isn't just lesbians and gay men who pay the bill. There are thoughtful observers who say the cost—from loss of productivity to the bills for stress, alcoholism, suicide—is in the billions. And how do you measure less visible costs like fear, anguish, and alienation? The cost, for example, to a family I know whose mother must call her son in secret; the father has forbidden all contact and has threatened to kill the son if he ever sees him.

If Kinsey's figures are close, there are at least fifteen million men and women in the United States whose adult sexual expression is more homosexual than heterosexual. Add their parents, and you have forty-five million people hurt by homophobia. It may be the last publicly acceptable bigotry. We have attempted to outlaw racism and sexism; the government is at least symbolically opposed. And science helped wipe out the ignorance that fueled them. But prejudice against lesbians and gay men is still okay in the capitols, the halls of ''justice,'' in the sanctuaries, the board rooms, and the laboratories.

This is likely to continue until science takes this human phenomenon seriously. Homophobia is too costly for us to remain ignorant. Knowledge alone won't end homophobia, but it's the essential first step.

It may be time for the surgeon general to commission the kind of studies the government fostered in other areas—from racism to the dangers of smoking. Time for science to send out a clear message: ''**Warning:** Homophobia may be dangerous to your society's health.''

PART FOUR

PUBLIC POLICY: WHEN SOCIETY IS THE PATIENT

Some bioethics dilemmas are intensely personal. In others, the decision is made by that vague entity called "society." These decisions are most clear when they're expressed in laws, regulations, or budgets. But sometimes they're just widely held attitudes, usually unquestioned because they're unseen. Here are some examples.

Murder, Mercy, or the Budget?

Are we in an epidemic of mercy killing? You probably remember a few highly publicized cases—for example, Roswell Gilbert, who shot his wife to death with a 9-mm handgun in March 1985, ending her seven years of suffering from Alzheimer's disease. Gilbert was seventy-six years old when he was sentenced to a life term. It was more than five years before the governor commuted his term and set him free.

It was the most publicized mercy killing in U.S. history—twenty months of news stories, interviews, courtroom sketches, minicam graphics, sermons, and editorials. NBC made a TV movie of it in 1988.

But concentrating on individual cases meant leaving out another dramatic development of the 1980s, one that puzzles and worries those who watch such things. It's the fact that mercy killing—the taking of a loved one's life to relieve suffering—increased dramatically during the decade.

Consider this:

In 1920 a Michigan court sentenced Frank Roberts to life in prison (and solitary confinement) for helping his terminally ill wife commit suicide. It was the first recorded prosecution for active euthanasia in the United States. In the next sixty-five years, through 1985, law enforcement agencies in this country handled sixty mercy-killing cases. Twenty of those cases, one-third of the total, occurred in one year: 1985. Nine others had been reported between 1980 and 1984, meaning twenty-nine of the sixty cases took place in the first half of the decade.

The results of those arrests in the early 1980s are also revealing: Besides Roswell Gilbert, only one of those twenty-nine people went to prison. Twenty-one were convicted of manslaughter but given suspended sentences or probation. Of the rest, two were acquitted, one was found not guilty because of temporary insanity, one case was dismissed by the judge, and in two there was no indictment.

One of the saddest cases was that of Dr. John Kraai, seventy-six, a much-beloved physician who was still making house calls in little Fairport, New York. One day he visited a long-time friend, eighty-one-year-old Fred Wagner, suffering in a nursing home from Alzheimer's disease and gangrene. When it was clear that Wagner recognized no one, and was in severe pain, Dr. Kraai injected him with a fatal dose of insulin. Arrested and freed on bail, aware that the district attorney intended to prosecute—and that Roswell Gilbert, his same age, had been sentenced to life a few months before—Dr. Kraai took his own life with an injection of Demerol.

Derek Humphrey thinks he knows why the number of mercy killings is growing. He's a co-founder of the Hemlock Society, the national organization working toward legal voluntary euthanasia for dying patients. But he's quick to say that "voluntary euthanasia and mercy killing are not the answer" to problems like Alzheimer's disease. "The picture [of mercy killers of Alzheimer's patients] is one of isolated existence, of loneliness and frustration," Humphrey says. "The lack of supportive care, not only for the patient but for the caregiver, is crucial."

In the strict sense, Roswell Gilbert's wife was not terminally ill. Nor was she in a coma. She couldn't recognize her husband and needed constant care, but she could have lived many more years. The problem was the hopelessness, the physical and emotional drain of being on duty twenty-four hours a day, 365 days a year.

Physicians, through ignorance or neglect, often fail to tell the family about groups like A.D., the Alzheimer's disease organization, that offer training, encouragement, and support.

"I talked to Gilbert in prison," Humphrey says. "He says none of the nurses or doctors ever suggested groups to whom he could go for help."

But why the increase in such tragedies?

"Across the country, as I travel to conferences, I hear one thing again and again. There no longer are funds for proper care of the sick and the elderly," Humphrey says.

The funds are drying up for affordable, acceptable nursing homes, enough visiting nurses, and community mental health programs. "I would speculate that if a proper study were done, it would show that a major factor in the increase in mercy killings is the government cutback in health funds" since 1980.

The picture of Roswell Gilbert in prison, facing his eightieth birthday, tears at the heart. It should also be a reminder of issues the rest of us would prefer to ignore. It might even force us to think about the budget priorities that deal so cruelly with those who love the sick and dying.

Our Chemistry Sets Go to War

Is chemical warfare morally wrong? Or morally wrong only when it's in the wrong hands? If that seems to be a dumb question, consider that the world's second greatest stockpiler of nerve gas, mustard gas, and other hellish chemical weapons is the United States. This fact hasn't been given much attention in the outbursts of concern that Iraq's Saddam Hussein has chemical weapons.

It's easy to forget that we abandoned President Nixon's 1969 moratorium on making chemical weapons after just a few years, and began adding to the tens of thousands of tons on hand. It's better not to think too hard about the hundreds of millions budgeted for research on "defensive" biological weapons.

We're not alone in having our universities and medical schools involved in this kind of research. Some of our enemies have poison gas; so do some of our allies. Some countries that have it were enemies yesterday and are friends today—and who knows what they'll be tomorrow?

But because I live in the United States, and love the country, I'm concerned that nobody is asking questions like these:

What is it about poison gas or germ warfare that makes them seem morally reprehensible? What does it do to the professions of science and medicine to be involved in developing these weapons?

Is it wrong for some nations and right for others? If so, what is the rationale? Without for a moment apologizing for the lunacy that dominates Libya, Iraq, or North Korea, it's fair to ask whether we have shown ourselves to be any more responsible. In negotiations in the late 1980s, we at first pushed for an outright, verifiable ban on chemical weapons—then backed off because U.S. manufacturers feared the loss of trade secrets.

Our government dumped Agent Orange on Vietnam and has

air-dropped toxic substances on our own citizens to see whether they worked. We bombed Libya—killing one of Colonel Gadhafi's small children—in retaliation for a terrorist act that later turned out to have been committed by Syria.

Dr. Keith Yamamoto, chair of biochemistry and biophysics at the University of California-San Francisco Medical School, says in his book *Gene Wars,*

> Every government engages in subterfuge to protect what it perceives as legitimate national security interests. To this end, over several decades, the Department of Defense and the CIA have systematically lied about, hidden, and disguised the range, depth, and goals of their chemical and biological warfare enterprises as well as the national policies on which they were based.
>
> In the process they have corrupted public and private institutions, sacrificed unwitting research subjects, and ignored serious public health and safety concerns.

Is poison gas worse than other weapons? Or do we fasten on it as a distraction from bigger weapons-control problems?

Is poison gas worse than the fire bombs the British dropped on Hamburg in World War II? The bombs were made of sticky phosphorus, which ignites when exposed to air. In *The Night Hamburg Died,* Martin Caidin tells of hundreds of civilians, unable to scrape the phosphorus from their bodies, standing neck-deep in the canals.

Once in a while someone would tentatively raise an arm out of the water, scream as it burst into flame, and pull it quickly back down. After three or four days, they slipped, one by one, beneath the water.

The lucky ones died instantly in fires that merged until the city was one fire, and the rising chimney of flame created a hundred-mile-an-hour hurricane of air rushing in from every direction.

Is chemical warfare worse?

Is it worse than our growing stockpile of biological agents, like genetically produced rattlesnake venom or cholera?

Is it worse than The Bomb?

My Uncle Jerry suffered for more than fifty years from the mustard gas he breathed as a seventeen-year-old Marine in the fields of France. That was 1917, and the "war to end all wars."

I suspect he would agree that the questions above are foolish and unanswerable, because the assumption behind them is wrong: that we can still justify any war.

So the Old Folks Are Killing Themselves Off

Well, the news is that the suicide rate among older people in the United States is soaring.

All through the 1980s, elderly Americans were killing themselves in growing numbers. In every other age group, the rate fell; even among teenagers, despite some widely publicized local problems, the suicide rate was down in the last half of the decade. So far in the 1990s, the trend hasn't changed.

Maybe the old folks are finally getting the message. Some countries venerate old age. But we make jokes about it (like that TV ad in which the silly old things can't remember the name of the restaurant). In some countries, older people live out their years in the bosom of their families, in the middle of the action, part of the lives of children and grandchildren. But we've isolated them, institutionalizing the separation in ghettoes that range from plush "retirement communities" to shabby residence hotels.

We've made it clear that a human being is most worthwhile at age twenty-five, when the skin is unwrinkled and the energy boundless. From there it's all downhill. And suicide is up among the elderly?

Some cultures think it's natural to see that older people have decent housing, enough food, and freedom from worry about medical costs—a way of paying back what they gave us. But we seem to consider near-poverty the norm for older people, and if a few of them have to eat canned dog food, they should be glad they live in a country where it's government-inspected.

To make sure they get the message, we rail at them for using up our Social Security money before we can get our hands on it. There is even a national lobby to wrest those oversize monthly payments from the oldsters. Hundreds of thousands of resentful baby boomers have joined. And we wonder that suicide is on the rise?

Do you suppose the old folks are finally realizing what society has been telling them for years: Peoples' worth is measured by what they produce, not by what kind of person they are? When they retire, they become an embarrassing and useless drain on the economy.

The strongest message we're sending them has to do with their fear of being sick, helpless, and broke before death comes. We're one of the very few industrial nations in the world that let elderly citizens bankrupt themselves trying to stay well. Trying to keep from being a burden on their children. We cut their Medicare health benefits while doctors' fees and hospital costs were going up, and then made them pay a bigger share of the cost. We made a big flourish about providing catastrophic health care, made the bill almost unworkable, and repealed it a year later.

Meanwhile, most discussion of the rising cost of health care

67

puts the blame on the elderly, especially those who take unreasonably long to die. The president could send a lot of younger folks to Mars with all that money.

All this encourages, among many older people, a sense of dread, a fear that independence and dignity are precarious luxuries that will be stripped away when we are too old to "deserve" them. Most industrial nations would have trouble understanding this. They seem to think simple justice requires guaranteeing at least decent shelter, food, and health care to older citizens. By refusing to do so, we've made our feelings pretty clear.

And yet the vast majority of older people don't get it. They insist on believing they are people of worth. They volunteer. They begin second careers. They baby-sit, go to school, or take up hobbies they didn't have time for when they were taking care of us. Most go about their daily lives with the same relative happiness and sense of purpose they had when they were younger. And 99,979 out of every 100,000 do not commit suicide.

Could it be that in their later years, they have gained some wisdom about life the rest of us don't have?

Sad Symbol of a National Problem

Estelle Browning lay in a nursing home bed in Clearwater, Florida, immobilized and semiconscious from a stroke. She was eighty-nine, and she wasn't aware that she had become a symbol for a statewide debate over the right to die. Her plight, and the arguments that swirled around her, remind us how complicated, how inconsistent, how confusing is our patchwork of ethical opinion and law on this subject.

Browning, like so many thoughtful people, used to worry about the possibility of ending up just this way—helpless in an institutional bed, her fate controlled by strangers. More than three years earlier she had drafted a "living will"—directing that she not be kept alive by artificial means if she wasn't able to give instructions. Then, within six months, came the stroke. Partly paralyzed, incommunicado, unable even to swallow, she was fitted with a tube to deliver nutrients and water to her stomach.

When it became clear that her condition wasn't likely to change for a while, they moved her to the Sunset Point Nursing Center. Her cousin and only relative, eighty-year-old Doris Herbert, had been made her legal guardian, and in March 1988 Herbert decided this had gone on long enough. She took the living will to court and asked that her cousin be allowed to die. She asked that the artificial feeding tube be removed.

But Circuit Court Judge Thomas Penick, Jr. refused the request. Doctors had testified at the hearing that Browning was not dying, and Florida law allowed patients to refuse food and water only if they are terminally ill. Herbert appealed, and a month later the Second District Court of Appeals overturned the lower court. The judges ruled unanimously that, as Browning's guardian, Herbert had the right to order the feeding tube removed.

By now the issue was being discussed in newspapers and on TV across Florida. So-called right-to-life groups got into the act, arguing against any removal of life support under any circumstances. Civil liberties groups argued for the historic right of patients to refuse treatment.

C. Marie King, the assistant state attorney for Pinellas-Pasco County, didn't like the appellate ruling and threatened to appeal. In her written argument she raised the specter of Hitler, killing the "useless" members of society. She wrote that it's morally wrong to remove feeding tubes in cases like this because it's "genocide of the elderly."

It isn't clear just how genocide could occur if the patient (or a chosen surrogate) makes the decision in each case. But it is an argument many people use.

Whether there was to be another appeal or not, Herbert said she would continue the fight. "This case and this issue won't go away," her lawyer told reporters. "For one Estelle Browning, there must be hundreds, if not thousands of people like her in Florida."

Herbert said: "I'm sorry that things turned out the way they did, that she had to suffer for two and a half years. I wanted more than anything for her to live (but) I also wanted her wishes carried out."

In July, the Florida Legislature passed a bill that would let people with living wills refuse life-support technology, including artificial feeding, if it wasn't helping the patient get better. Governor Bob Martinez vetoed it.

A few days later, there was another development in the case. Estelle Browning died of natural causes. She was alone, still connected to the feeding tube.

Time for Us to Get into the Game

"Politics," said Aristotle, "is ethics writ large."

Over the past few years you could see them writing, turning ethical issues into legislation. With smoke and mirrors, with common sense and wishful thinking, with prayer and pragmatism and press conferences, the process went on.

An example was surrogate motherhood. The California Assembly passed a bill that would outlaw "surrogate mother" contracts, under which women are paid to bear children for infertile couples. It was no coincidence that the vote came the same day as an emotion-laden, made-for-TV movie about the surrogate mother who changed her mind and refused to give up the baby. The legislatures of twenty-five other states considered bills about surrogate mothering. Of the first three states to pass laws, Arkansas calls the contracts valid, while Louisiana and Nebraska forbid them.

The National Coalition Against Surrogacy joined the ''ethics writ large'' endeavor, holding a press conference one day in Washington. It was led by Baby M's birth-mother, described unfortunately by the Associated Press as ''landmark surrogate Mary Beth Whitehead . . .''

The Coalition's agenda, its leaders said, was putting the ''baby brokers'' out of business. Such brokers, usually lawyers, bring infertile couples together with women willing to bear a child. Their fee is usually equal to the fee of the birth-mother—around $10,000. ''We want this surrogacy industry gone,'' said Gena Corea in a speech. ''Let it stop feeding off our flesh.''

Lobbying in California, but not invited to the Washington event, were the 10 to 20 percent of American married couples who want babies and can't have them. Their desperation is reflected in figures from a recent government report: They spend $1 billion a year trying to get pregnant, including $70 million on in-vitro fertilization—the still-experimental ''test-tube baby'' procedure.

The fears of infertile couples were voiced by a legislator who said banning surrogate mothering would ''create more misery and hopelessness in the lives of people who want children'' but are physically unable to produce their own children.

While rhetoric, stridency, and a touch of show-biz are traditional in the business of turning ethics into public policy, there's an element missing here: thoughtful, widespread debate by the public. More than gut reactions and instinctive leaps to one side or the other, we need to be asking questions such as these:

• Is it innately wrong for a woman to have a baby for a childless couple? Would it be different if it were done free—for a relative, for example, rather than for money?

• Would it be acceptable if the couple were not infertile, but simply wanted to avoid interrupting her career?

• What ideals and traditions form our attitude toward having—or not having—children? Is involuntary childlessness a disease? If it is, should it be "cured" at any cost? What drives us to have our "own" child?

• What does it mean to "have" a child? Is it ownership? Guardianship? Stewardship?

• How is surrogate mothering different from other adoptions? Is there an element of judgment in some opposition to fertility measures—a vague belief that the couple is childless because they deserve to be punished? Is there a stigma attached because much infertility is caused by sexually transmitted diseases?

• Why hasn't more money been spent on research to prevent infertility?

• What is the role of law in such private matters? What is the minimum law we could pass and still protect all the parties?

You should be asking these questions, and many more of your own. They should be asked in public and private, anywhere issues are discussed. We're talking about human lives, infant and adult, and the subject is far too important to be left to the lawyers, legislators, doctors, and bioethicists.

PART FIVE
THE NEW REPRODUCTION: TURMOIL IN (AND OUT OF) THE WOMB

*I*t was scientists who raised the dilemma, by learning to fertilize human eggs in the laboratory and store them indefinitely by freezing. But science could do little to solve the problem: What to do with the seven frozen embryos stored by Junior and Mary Sue Davis before their marriage fell apart?

In Tennessee, Judge W. Dale Young had to decide whether Mary Sue should have control of the seven tiny embryos—visible only through a microscope—she and Junior had stored in a freezer in Knoxville as part of a six-year struggle to have a baby.

The embryos resulted from in-vitro fertilization (IVF), which involved extracting eggs from Mary Sue's ovaries and fertilizing them in a laboratory dish with Junior's sperm. IVF was a last-chance end run around Mary Sue's blocked fallopian tubes. The marriage went bad before the embryos could be implanted in her womb, but Mary Sue still wanted a child. Junior Davis said no; he no longer wanted to cooperate with Mary Sue in anything, especially having a baby. The embryos were as much his as hers, he told the divorce judge, and he wanted them left in storage. Deciding what to do with the embryos was to be the last step in the divorce settlement.

It was a classic case for the relatively new discipline called bioethics, the study of unexpected side effects of the biological revolution. It's a social, ethical, or legal dilemma created by advances in biology or medicine—brought on by science, but not solvable by science.

Here are some of the more intriguing questions behind the Davises' dilemma:

• Are the embryos human beings? "They have already been

fertilized,'' Mary Sue told the court, ''and to me that is the beginning of life. Putting them in storage indefinitely, that's killing them.''

Her belief that life is human from the moment of fertilization—a belief that is not uncommon among the public—determines her attitude toward the seven microscopic dots. Her attorney even brought in an IVF expert to testify that other parents-to-be, seeing their embryos through a microscope, are ''usually very excited,'' and speak of them as they would of a newborn baby.

• What to do with the other embryos? Mary Sue didn't say what she would do with the four or five she didn't plan to use. Not leave them stored indefinitely, of course; that would be murder. Pour them down the drain? Pull the plug on the freezer? For her, the ''human at fertilization'' theory raised as many problems as it solved.

Junior Davis didn't directly challenge the theory, but used a word in court obviously intended to define the objects in question in a different manner: ''I oppose the use of the pre-embryos. . . .''

• Is childlessness a disease, to be cured at any cost? In a society that pushes every couple to have children, being barren can be agony. True, this is changing, and couples have more of a choice, but if you want kids, inability to have them is serious.

• But what is a legitimate cost, in emotion and energy and burden to the health care system? There are dozens of IVF clinics around the world; the original one alone has helped more than a thousand couples to have babies. But for each success there were nine failures, and IVF represents only a fraction of the health care effort spent on fertility.

• Who has the right to make this decision? In abortion debates, location affects the argument; the embryo is inside the woman's body and, after a few days, attached to it. It seems natural that the woman should decide.

But the Davis embryos were in Knoxville, fifteen miles up U.S. 129 from the courtroom in Maryville, not in Mary Sue's womb. Did this make them less completely Mary Sue's, and give her husband at least an equal share? The judge said no, giving "custody" to Mary Sue, but it could have gone either way.

• What if the embryos were just left in storage? Consider this possibility: Seventy years from now, long after the Davises have died, a lawyer informs distant relatives that they have inherited the frozen embryos. They sell the embryos to a childless couple, and the wife bears a child.

Junior and Mary Sue Davis are parents at last.

What to Do About Abuse in the Womb?

It's one of the toughest riddles in a time filled with health-care riddles: What to do about the pregnant woman whose acts endanger the fetus she's carrying. It's more complex than simply mother versus fetus or civil liberties versus the duty to protect the helpless.

• In Laramie, Wyoming, Diane Pfannenstiel, four months pregnant, was arrested for violating a judge's order not to drink while she was pregnant. She had a blood alcohol level high enough to be "intoxicated" under state law, and was charged with felony child abuse. But the judge dismissed the charge, saying the state hadn't proved that the fetus had been injured.

• In Michigan a judge ordered Kimberly Hardy to stand trial for child abuse and "delivering cocaine"—a charge usually used against dealers—to her baby boy. The judge avoided the touchy question of whether the fetus was actually a human being by ruling that the cocaine was delivered during the seconds after the baby had been born, but before the umbilical cord was cut.

• A Florida judge jailed a woman for six days for having intercourse with her husband in defiance of a doctor who had told her it would endanger the fetus.

There is general agreement on one thing: Fetal abuse is a serious problem. It may be growing, with widespread use of drugs like alcohol and cocaine, and the growing numbers of young women with HIV—the virus that can cause AIDS in their babies.

The heated disagreement is over what to do about the problem. Some favor taking control of the woman's life, either by jail or enforced hospitalization. They say the devastating impact of abuse in the womb goes on and on: crack babies, even after physical rehabilitation, are having so many severe emotional problems and exhibit such uncontrollable behavior that elementary schools are having to segregate many of them.

In the introduction to Michael Dorris's moving book *The Broken Cord,* Louise Erdrich, adoptive mother of three children with fetal alcohol syndrome, says:

> I would rather have been incarcerated for nine months and produce a normal child than bear a human being who would, for the rest of his or her life, be imprisoned by what I had done.
>
> If you don't agree with me, then go and sit beside the alcohol-affected while they try to learn how to add. Dry their frustrated tears. . . . Hold their heads when they have unnecessary seizures and wipe the blood from their bitten lips. . . . Watch them suffer a crime they won't understand committing.''

Those who favor incarceration also argue that the threat would make mothers-to-be less likely to use drugs. And they point out that even *Roe vs. Wade,* the historic pro-choice ruling, doesn't give a woman absolute power over a fetus in the last three months of pregnancy.

On the other side are those who fear that a policy of incarceration could make a mother liable for anything that goes wrong with a pregnancy. They ask where the law would draw the line. Overeating—also known to have its impact? Less than perfect control of blood sugar by a diabetic, with the resulting risk of birth defects? Exercising too much? Not exercising at all?

They also argue that fear of the police could cause women to avoid much-needed prenatal visits. And they believe that the costs to the civil rights of pregnant women would be too high. Barbara Katz Rothman has written: "We are in danger of creating of pregnant women a second class of citizen, without basic legal rights or bodily integrity and self-determination."

Attorney Jane Gallagher has written of "the recurrent temptations to view and treat pregnant women as vessels."

How would you handle the problem?

If there is a middle way in all this, it has to be a strong and effective program of education available to all potential mothers. Unfortunately, this is like so many other health areas: We'd rather deal with the awful results than get serious about prevention.

One Thing We Know About Abortion

It may be impossible, amid the cannons' roar and smoke, to be rational about Supreme Court decisions on abortion. But let's try.

Let's take one little piece of the religious-political-medical-social puzzle, and remind ourselves of one thing we know for

77

sure. We know for sure that science doesn't tell us what it is to be human.

Look at the man lying in the intensive-care unit, unresponsive, on full life support. Is he human? Is there a reason we fall back on the word *vegetable* and the doctors use *persistent vegetative state*? If he has any brain activity left, he's alive. If he hasn't, he is a corpse, even though the machines keep air and blood flowing through his body.

Medicine didn't make that decision. The state legislatures defined, in the light of new technology, the difference between life and death in this case.

We know that down through history there have been many definitions of humanity. We don't die all at once; the organs give up at different rates. So some clergy made a decision: Death occurs a certain number of minutes after the heart stops. A more secular decision comes from a coroner who makes society's decision. He or she estimates when the body reached a certain arbitrarily chosen temperature. That, officially, is when the person died.

Was Ferdinand Marcos alive during the weeks he lay in the intensive care unit, his kidneys dead, his mind permanently asleep, his lungs and heart working only because of artificial support? If he was alive, it was because his wife considered him alive and his doctors treated him as though he were, not because there's some sort of scientific scale that tells us so. So it is, believe it or not, at the other end of life.

If you think humanity means having a soul, there isn't any spectrometer or radiation counter that tells when the soul enters the embryo or fetus. If the "soul" is a meaningless concept to you, you still must decide at what time the embryo or fetus—potentially human—becomes fully so.

Recent Supreme Court rulings seem to encourage the

suggestion that the embryo is fully human from the second of fertilization. That's a commonly held belief. So is the belief that humanity doesn't come until there are eight cells and the tiny speck has attached to the mother's body. Some strains of Judaism said the embryo becomes human sixty days after fertilization—if it is male. Ninety days for females.

One of the most popular theories has been that humanity is present when the mother-to-be first feels the fetus move—technically, "quickening." The vast majority of induced abortions take place in the four months or so before quickening. Until 1869 the Roman Catholic Church didn't prohibit abortions before the woman could feel the fetus move.

The 1972 Supreme Court decision, besides saying that the state has no business dictating women's reproductive decisions, gave implied consent to another theory: that the fetus is really human when it no longer has to rely on the mother's body for life. That would be around six months.

These theories have one thing in common: Not one of them is scientifically provable. The decision has to be a moral one.

A Question About the Abortion Debate

You can't help wondering whether the abortion debate isn't really about women, not fetuses. The arguments over whether a fetus is fully human may have diverted us from a prior question: In our society, is a woman fully a human being?

If you think that's a dumb question, consider this: For nine years the U.S. House of Representatives voted against funding abortions for poor women impregnated through rape or incest. In 1989, when such funding finally passed, 209 representatives voted against. They knew that if they prevailed again, thousands of poor women would be forced to complete pregnancies they didn't want.

Whether you agree with the anti-abortion vote or not, it's hard to ignore the message behind the vote: A woman was less valuable, less "human" than a fetus. There's more to the message. When a girl is sexually molested by a father or older brother, she's often the one who gets blamed.

And rape? In Florida, a jury acquitted an accused rapist—a man wanted in Georgia on numerous other rape counts—because the victim had dressed "provocatively." Experts believe that only one in ten rapes gets reported, and that the reason is the woman's societally induced guilt and the fear that she'll be blamed.

We're talking not about individual acts, but a system's approach to hatred—attitudes integral to our way of life. A few homely examples:

• When somebody pointed out, a few years back, that the Mormon Church had refused to ordain blacks as priests, a self-righteous press jumped all over them. The news media wouldn't let go of the story until church policy changed. Nobody ever mentioned that the Mormons, like many other denominations, barred priesthood to a much bigger oppressed group: women.

• Those who study homophobia suggest that the most passionate element in hatred of gays is directed at the "poisoning" of males by a strong feminine component. It's okay for a girl to be a tomboy, but not for a boy to be a sissy. Do you think it's just an accident of culture that women can wear pants in public but men can't wear dresses?

• Doctors still perform with impunity far more Cesarean sections and hysterectomies than are medically justified. It's not such a big deal; the subjects are women.

• The policy of a national news service is to speak of a Supreme Court justice, after once giving the full name, as "Justice Rehnquist." Except, of course, Sandra Day O'Connor. She's "Mrs. O'Connor." An Army major: "Miss" or "Mrs. Jones." A police sergeant: "Mrs. Elson." Language not only expresses our thoughts; it helps define them, and as a people we doggedly resist making our language more gender-inclusive. Despite the inclusion of women in Jesus' ministry and the leadership of the early church, a large segment of Christianity goes into shock at the idea of inclusive language.

The point is not that there is bigotry, but that it is systemic—so thoroughly a part of our way of life that we don't see it unless somebody points it out. Individual hatred may make a man commit rape; systemic hatred is the "folk wisdom" that lets him off because the woman was to blame.

President Bush's attempted veto of those funds Congress voted for victims of rape and incest meant the government still believed in enforced pregnancy. Writer Larry Letich points out that unwanted pregnancy is best compared with unwanted sex. Freely chosen, sex and pregnancy can be wonderful. Unwanted sex, forced sex, is called rape. Forced pregnancy? It's government policy. Letich says, "As difficult as it may be morally for some people to accept abortion, there is a greater wrong—a greater immorality—in forcing a woman to undergo experiences as demanding, intimate, and at times life-threatening as pregnancy and childbirth."

Do you think it would be happening if it were men who bore the babies?

PART SIX
AIDS: A CHALLENGE TO US ALL

---

*I*t is the most frightening plague since the deadly days of polio in the 1950s. It has forced improvements in medical research and in health education. It has triggered massive expressions of concern and compassion, and encouraged expressions of bigotry as violent as those of the lynching days. It is exposing the inadequacies of our patchwork health care system. And by confronting us with complex moral and social decisions, it is reminding us that bioethics is no longer a spectator sport.

Why Ryan Made Us So Afraid

Ryan White's death in April 1990 was a reminder of how willing we are to abandon our historic ideals of justice and compassion. You remember Ryan's story: At thirteen he was infected with HIV, the AIDS-causing virus, through a clotting agent, a blood product, he took for hemophilia. When the word of his infection got out, he was hounded from school and eventually from Kokomo, his home town.

He was one of at least 10,000 hemophiliacs infected with HIV before we learned how to screen the blood and purify the clotting agent. Like Ryan, hundreds went on to develop symptoms of AIDS, and like him, many have suffered hatred and injustice.

The three little Ray brothers, all hemophiliacs, were barred from their elementary school in Florida after testing positive for HIV. Mobs surrounded their house, and later it was burned to the ground. The Rays left town.

It wasn't just the Midwest and South, either. In trendy Carmel,

California, nine-year-old Ben Oyler was barred from classes because so many parents objected. Months later, after he died, his mother told reporters: "That rejection, for a little boy to have to take that, it's pretty sad there aren't more understanding hearts."

All the more sad because anybody who bothers to check it out knows that no one has ever been infected with HIV from casual contact. A 1989 study of more than fifty families where one child was HIV-positive failed to find a single cause of spread to another family member—not even those who shared toothbrushes.

Why is it there are so few understanding hearts out there? What turned the young parents of Carmel into a snarling, panicky pack, hounding a dying third-grader? It's not just that AIDS is a fatal disease. There are germs and viruses out there more easily caught, and just as deadly. The real reasons are deeper in our collective psyche.

We're afraid, because we're afraid of sex. The subject frightens us into silence, or into bad jokes. And AIDS is mostly a sexually transmitted disease. And since humans first identified sexually transmitted diseases, they have been seen as a special threat to civilization. They endangered our heritage, threatening our survival as peoples—by making women sterile or making the babies fatally sick. These primal fears disappeared within a generation when we found cures for diseases like gonorrhea and syphilis. But in 1981 we suddenly again faced an epidemic disease, usually sexually transmitted, that could kill the offspring of infected women.

We're afraid because we're afraid of homosexuality. AIDS is not a "gay" disease; most of the people in the world infected with HIV are women and children. It happened that in the United States it was first introduced among gays, and its sexual transmission was to other gays. But AIDS is still seen, almost universally in the United States, as an affliction of homosexuals. If you doubt this, look up the graffiti painted on the Ray kids' house or scrawled by fellow students on Ryan's locker: "Faggot!" "Queer!"

Never mind that the infections of Ryan White and the Florida boys had nothing to do with sex. We're a society in which homophobia—some call it heterosexism—is woven into the fabric of life. Reared from birth on "homo" jokes, we're like the people raised to put down blacks or women: It takes a conscious effort to overcome our bigotry—and the fear behind it.

We're afraid because we think AIDS is a punishment from God. Never mind that the leaders of the major denominations, from United Methodist to Roman Catholic, have rejected such an idea. The fact is that we subconsciously feel blame.

So what do we do? Historians say that in killer epidemics, societies always look for a scapegoat. By killing, exiling, or blaming one specific group, we always hope to deflect the lightning bolt, distracting attention from the rest of us and purifying the majority so we won't be punished any more. It's no coincidence that some of the worst persecution of Jews in Europe came during the great plagues.

At the time of Ryan's widely publicized death, the civic leaders of Kokomo were assuring the country that his troubles could have happened anywhere, and that only a handful of Kokomo people were involved in the harassment. They may be right on the first point—although Ryan and his mother did immediately find another town and a school where he had a warm welcome. Wrong on the second point. Everybody in Kokomo was involved, either actively helping the White family or, by their silence, joining the baying pack.

So were the rest of us, and will be the next time fear chases justice and compassion away. As Edmund Burke said: ''All that is required for evil to triumph is that good [people] do nothing.''

Has AIDS Destroyed Our Brains?

Come on, folks, let's beam back down to earth. It's time for a dose of reality. As a news junkie and sometime sociologist, I've been fascinated with the weird and the bizarre ever since pilot Douglas ''Wrong-way'' Corrigan took off from a New York airport heading for Los Angeles and ended up in Ireland. But I haven't seen anything to compare with our abandonment of rational thought in the AIDS crisis.

Here we are in the midst of a serious epidemic, calling for cool heads, objectivity, and clear communication. Instead, we've pushed the panic button. We're babbling gibberish. We're willing to spend money, sacrifice civil liberties, suspend all critical judgment, and lock up our neighbors if it will just keep the AIDS bug from pouncing on us.

It's not just the ''Dukes of Hazzard'' crowd. From doctors to governors, from sheriffs to TV evangelists, we seem to have gone into a mental twilight zone, where feelings and fears take precedence over facts.

Take the biters, for example. As I write this, there are at least ten HIV-infected people in jails across the country facing charges of attempted murder for biting peace officers. One of them, serving five years for armed robbery, has just been sentenced to life on an attempted murder charge because he bit a prison guard.

Think about it for a moment. It's nine years into the epidemic, and scientists feel confident in ruling out tears and saliva as carriers of HIV. There isn't enough of the virus present to matter, and nobody is known to have been infected by these fluids.

You can't *give* somebody the AIDS virus by biting them. On the other hand, you can *get* HIV by biting somebody! An infected person's blood does carry the virus, and if the blood gets in your mouth while you have a sore or cut there, you could be infected. So if it's spread through biting at all, it would be the biters who are in danger, not the bitees!

Understand: I'm not condoning assaults with the teeth or any other part of the body. But I hope I'm demonstrating how silly we can be amid the panic over AIDS. Responsible people—juries and sheriffs, for example—can be driven by public panic to acts that have no connection to reality and that do nothing to stop the AIDS epidemic.

A more serious example is the proposal for mandatory testing. Public health experts, from the last two surgeon generals to most AIDS prevention workers, have pointed out that forced testing would not only be prohibitively expensive, but wouldn't get the job done because it would drive those most at risk underground. But the list of people who want to impose such tests goes right to the top of the organizational chart.

Another serious example: Former Interior Secretary James Watt was heard asking college students in Oregon, "Do you want an AIDS victim to sneeze on your salad?" To save our salads, Watt endorsed a solution often proposed: Not only force HIV testing, but use isolation camps to lock up everybody who has the virus. Given Watt's record of ethnic slurs and foot-in-mouth disease, it would be easy enough to dismiss him as another loose cannon. Except for one thing: Millions of our fellow citizens agree with him.

They favor "quarantine"—unaware of its scope and cost—not just for the 50,000 or so with AIDS, but for the one to two million HIV carriers who are equally infectious, through sex or exchange of blood. They persist, despite proof that education has stopped the spread of new cases of HIV infection in one target community—gay men—without locking anybody up.

Support for quarantine is a phenomenon not fully explained by the passion to isolate a scapegoat, or by the need for a simplistic quick fix, or by our willingness to toss the Bill of Rights overboard in any scary emergency, or even by systemic homophobia. But put all these emotional issues together and they're a powerful force. That's why I believe we are in real danger, before this epidemic is over, of ''interning'' as many HIV carriers as we can.

Fear will do it, just as racism, overriding logic and the Bill of Rights, imprisoned Japanese-Americans in 1942. That was bad enough. But we exposed our real ideals when we let German-Americans, because they were white, stay free.

Is AIDS Getting Too Much Money?

Is AIDS getting more than its share of federal funding? Many people think so. They point out that the government in 1990 spent about as much on AIDS, which had killed just 75,000 people in ten years, as it did on cancer, which killed 500,000 Americans that year alone. Heart disease got only about two-thirds as much, and it took another 750,000 citizens in 1989.

But people who look at the whole health care scene are warning us that this kind of comparison is irrelevant—and could be dangerous. In the first place, the problems are vastly different. As our population ages, cancer and heart disease will increase somewhat. But AIDS is exploding: 75,000 had died, but 263,000 were expected to die in the next three years.

There is barely hospital or nursing-home space for the AIDS patients we have now, medical economists say. While insurance companies and the federal government debate who should pay, hospitals in the major cities already are stretched beyond limits, facing bankruptcy, with depleted and burned-out staffs. This endangers everybody who might need a hospital bed someday.

The whole health care system is being put to the test by this epidemic in a way no other health problem has. Restricting funding because of a misguided "fairness" test will hurt us all, not just those with HIV. Pitting disease against disease distracts us from the real issues—sort of like fighting for deck-chair space on the *Titanic*.

It keeps us from considering how to hold down health costs, which are rising four times as fast as inflation. It lets us ignore the growing demand that everybody should have at least a minimum guaranteed access to health care.

It distracts us from questioning the misguided assumptions on which our health care system is built.

It keeps us from noticing the advances in immunology, community-based care, rapid new-drug approval, and hospice care that have emerged during the crisis.

Pointing to AIDS as overfunded is popular, sociologists say, because those most at risk for AIDS are people already stigmatized, especially gay men, needle-using drug addicts, and prostitutes. A Canadian health minister justified his country's slow response to AIDS by saying it was a "self-inflicted disease; they shot themselves in the foot." But health professionals point out that the vast majority of the people dying of AIDS at that time, in 1989, had been infected before anybody knew the virus existed, or how it was spread.

They point out vastly different attitudes toward people with cancer and heart attacks. The words *irresponsible* or *undeserving* don't come up—despite wide agreement that a high percentage of these tragedies are caused by smoking, overeating, and lack of exercise.

Smoking killed more than 350,000 Americans in 1989. Nobody talked about "self-inflicted" deaths or of patients shooting themselves in the foot. For that matter, health economists say well over half of all the burden of illness in this country is preventable. If that's so, it means that we waste, on avoidable ills, some $250 billion a year—a quarter of a trillion dollars. Now that, an objective observer might say, is a figure worth worrying about.

PART SEVEN
THE CHANGING FACE OF DEATH

*L*ounging on Bill's backyard deck on a Saturday morning, we used to wax glibly philosophical about everything from playing first base to the meaning of the Dead Sea Scrolls.

Mike the college teacher, George the school superintendent, Bill the Madison Avenue advertising salesman, and Bruce the bioethicist. On Saturday mornings we could let down our guard, drop the professional armor, and reveal some of the inner person. We could also disagree endlessly, debating the unsolvable while the coffee got cold.

It was around the time that Karen Ann Quinlan's family was fighting to free her from her permanent coma, and the subject of death came up several times. We were certain about our deaths; in rare unanimity, we all wanted to go fast. No lingering, no suffering.

Bill was a handsome man, built like a fullback. He had the outward confidence it took to walk into an office and sell a dozen advertisement pages in *Family Circle* magazine at $30,000 a page. When he arrived at a party, the center of focus changed, flowing around him.

But his heart was in La Mancha, not Manhattan. He quit for a while and moved to Greece so he could savor its color and history. Kicked out by the right-wing colonels' junta, he was lured back into selling, and quit again to teach high school English literature, at one-quarter the money. He believed teaching was a whole lot more important.

Other than my wife, Virginia, he was my best friend. He and I shared the chronic romantics' love for the play *Cyrano de Bergerac,* and—at least on Saturday mornings—could admit we got a lump in our throats every time we read that last act: Cyrano reporting the news to Roxanne, ending with the casual announcement of his own mortal wound and the reminder of his unshaken integrity: "My white plume!"

Bill had beaten cancer twice. One bout took a kidney; the second took one eye. He handled it all with a wry grin. The night before the eye operation, he took an eyebrow pencil and drew a big arrow pointing to the eye to be removed: "This one!!" Later, he was inclined to raise a coffee cup, fix us with his glass eye and intone, "Here's looking at you, kid!"

I moved across the continent and didn't see Bill till I went back to officiate at his wedding to Lynn. Just a few months later, I heard from a friend that the cancer was back, although Bill hadn't bothered to mention it in our phone calls. The details mostly came second-hand; eventually he had to quit his job, but then seemed to be getting stronger.

I was at a computer terminal one morning when a call came.

"Hey, this is Bill! George and Mike and I are sitting here planning my funeral, and we want you to come out here and be a part of it.

"When? Oh, in about two weeks. Why, you in a hurry? Anyway, do you think you can get away?"

In the days that followed, I heard about Bill's life as it wound down. He had long talks with his children from his first marriage, three of them teen-agers, and for the first time in years was able to say to each, "I love you, you know." He made some sense out of his tangled financial affairs. He called in a half-dozen people with whom he'd had words over the years: "I want you to know I've forgiven you, and I hope you've forgiven me." He savored the luxury of frankness, of not holding back. His last hours with Lynn were the richest of their seventeen-month marriage.

I talked with him the night before he died, his voice strained and faint across 3,000 miles. "It's tough, but I'm glad I didn't go fast,'' he said. ''There's been time to say good-bye to the people I love, and to set things right with a lot of people.

''I'm glad you can't see me; I'm not much to look at now, and I can't get out of bed anymore. But there's one thing the Big C can't take away: 'My white plume.' ''

Facing the Unanswerable Question

For nine years they had taken care of their father, and now they were being asked whether they wanted to hasten his death. Ever since a stroke had left him half-paralyzed, the two men had adjusted their careers and family life to his needs. A month at a time, one of the sons would move into his house.

During the day there was a paid helper, but at other times they read to him, watched television with him, helped him shuffle to the bathroom, bathed him, and tucked him into bed. He had been alert and responsive, but couldn't say a word. Now they were thinking about cutting off his food and water. Their father had been brought into the hospital two weeks earlier, after a new stroke, and was put on a ventilator to help him breathe.

''He kept trying to tell us something with his eyes,'' the older son said. ''We knew what it was: He wanted us to let him go. But we didn't want to hear it.''

They talked to the doctor, who said he would follow their wishes. ''We can do a full-court press if you want, even though there is no medical indication that he can recover. We can wait for the pneumonia, and choose then whether to treat it or not. Or we can turn off the ventilator now.''

The brothers talked—in the hospital cafeteria, in their father's strangely empty kitchen late at night. When they could talk logically, they agreed. It was their emotions that made the decision so difficult. Grudgingly, during that week, they concluded that the thing their father seemed to want was the thing they should do.

"We knew we couldn't take care of him at home any longer, not in this condition. And we kept remembering the way he had talked about Karen Ann Quinlan, saying he never wanted to end up living on tubes that way. We came to feel that the real act of love would be to let him go. After a week, we agreed to have the respirator turned off. When we made the decision, we suddenly realized it was the right thing to do. We called the doctor right away."

But it was too late. Turning off the ventilator was no longer one of their choices. Their father didn't need the breathing support any more. He still lay there, unresponsive, unmoving, fed through a hole in his stomach, but subtle body changes had made him able to breathe on his own.

For a moment, the sons were elated . . . and then helpless and discouraged. There was no hope this would lead to recovery. And the decision they had reached with such difficulty was meaningless.

For a time there had been a choice, and now the choice was gone. The next time they saw the doctor, he told them there was another choice: Stop the artificial feeding.

"We had to go through the whole emotional process again. But this time it was harder. Turning off an artificial machine is one thing. Cutting off his food and water is quite another."

Ten years ago it was Quinlan and several other cases about ventilators. By the time that became generally acceptable, there was a new round of difficult decisions—about withdrawing artificial feeding.

Now more than a dozen state courts have said that artificial feeding is medical treatment and can be withdrawn under certain conditions. The AMA took a stand in 1986 that artificial feeding is the same as ventilator support. Across the country, doctors are accepting the idea, but slowly. And there are still many who feel it's wrong to stop feeding a patient, no matter how ill.

The brothers agonized for a few more days, and then called the doctor.

"Doc? Hi, we've come to a decision," the brother on the phone said.

Who Speaks for the Living Dead?

She was the Karen Ann Quinlan of the 1980s. Like Karen, whose name was on every tongue in 1976, Nancy Cruzan lay on her side, her tense muscles drawing her into a fetal curl. Like Karen in her last six or seven years, Nancy breathed on her own, and sometimes opened her eyes. But—also like Karen—she saw nothing, didn't respond to noise or touch, and was in a vegetative state so deep that she wouldn't ever respond.

She'd been that way since a car accident six years ago. Like Karen's parents, Nancy's wanted to stop the life support—in this case, by removing a tube that delivers nutrition and liquids through a hole in her stomach.

And like Karen, Nancy Cruzan was at the center of a court battle likely to affect all of us.

But as the U.S. Supreme Court heard arguments, it was clear that some issues were different this time around. For example:

• **Withdrawing food and water.** The issue for the Quinlans was removing a breathing machine on which Karen seemed dependent. When it turned out she could breathe on her own after all, they didn't question the remaining artificial support: the nutrition and liquids necessary for life, as well as antibiotics given for continual infections.

Nancy's parents argue, in line with several states' court rulings, that artificial feeding is more like medical care than like a cup of soup, and withdrawing it is as morally acceptable as turning off the respirator.

• **The anti-abortion movement.** In Karen's day the anti-choice movement had little clout, and its activists hadn't yet identified "death and dignity" for adults as a concept that could weaken their defense of the fetus. Now, drawing power from direct lines to the White House, the movement is a major factor in any dispute involving decisions between life and death.

• **The conservative Supreme Court.** This was the first time the U.S. Supreme Court had accepted a "right to die" case, after refusing four other cases, including Karen's.

• **Rights of the disabled.** Several organizations that fight discrimination against the disabled filed briefs against the Cruzans. One of these says, "Ms. Cruzan has a disability. Her family seeks to withdraw food and fluids not because Ms. Cruzan is dying, but because she will live disabled."

Some of the issues haven't changed:

• **The quasi-judicial power of doctors.** Two-thirds of the country's physicians say they have been involved in decisions like the Cruzans'. In thousands of cases, the parents' wishes were respected. But if a doctor (or hospital administration) disagrees, he or she has the power to make a court case of it. The motives for this are never simple and can vary widely, from the conviction that withdrawal is wrong all the way to fear of lawsuits, fear of death, or an awe of technology.

• **Autonomy versus the public good.** Missouri's state attorneys argued that the state's interest in defending life is absolute; the parents said health care decisions for their daughter are part of keeping the government off one's back.

• **The dilemma of proxy consent.** The toughest problem is this: "How do you presume to speak for one who can't speak for herself? And who should speak?" It isn't enough to say that it's impossible to speak for someone else. Not making a decision is the same as making a decision.

In June 1990 the Court ruled against the Cruzans and for Missouri. Saying states had a right to specify the level of evidence required for withdrawing life-sustaining treatment of a comatose patient, the Court, however, affirmed the right of a competent patient or a surrogate to refuse treatment, even if it means death. And, surprisingly, it drew no distinction between artificial feeding and other forms of life support.

A Murder with No Killer

A young father was charged with murder in Chicago, but he was not the real killer. And fifteen-month-old Sammy, who died in his father's arms, was not the victim.

Twenty-three-year-old Rodolfo Linares pulled a gun and ordered a nurse out of the pediatric intensive-care unit, where Sammy had lain for eight months in a persistent vegetative state, breathing only with mechanical help. Rodolfo disconnected the ventilator and sat crying with Sammy in his arms until the boy died. Then he handed over his gun and submitted to arrest. He was charged with first-degree murder.

But the crucial event in the short life of Samuel Linares didn't take place that day. It happened eight months earlier, after Sammy was brought into the hospital, blue and unconscious from lack of oxygen. Something, a balloon or a piece of foil, was caught in his throat.

It wasn't clear how long he'd been without oxygen. But doctors know that the brain begins to die as quickly as four minutes after oxygen is cut off. This irreversible decay begins at the front of the brain, where judgment, speech, and critical thought reside, and moves back toward the base of the brain. Last to die, this bundle of nerves controls the automatic functions, like breathing.

Little Sammy was far enough gone that there were no signals to the chest muscles; he couldn't breathe on his own. Then came the crucial event: The emergency-room team, according to one account, worked twelve hours—*twelve hours*—to get him stabilized and breathing on the ventilator.

He lay like that for eight months, while his parents agonized over the news that he could live on this way for many years, and regularly asked the doctors to free him. The doctors told the father that if Sammy's brain had been completely gone, Illinois law would let them turn off the respirator. In California, as in many other states, courts have ruled that it can be legal to withdraw life support. But Illinois' Supreme Court is considering two such cases; until it rules, many doctors aren't going to stick their necks out.

"No one has the right to take the law into his own hands," the Cook County state's attorney said. Most of us would agree with that statement. But some of us would ask if that isn't just what the doctors did in the extraordinary effort that "saved" Sammy eight months earlier. There is no law requiring such an all-out attempt. It's a judgment call. How hard a physician works to resuscitate a patient depends on many things—mainly, the likelihood of recovery and the quality of life afterward.

But doctors are human, and sometimes other factors take over.

97

These factors may well be the real culprits in the case of Sammy Linares: fear of lawsuits, inability to deal with death, institutional rigidity, and even the need for medical students to get experience.

And the victims? Not Sammy, who wasn't suffering and is now free. But there were others:

The nurse, left forever with the memory of a loaded .357 Magnum in her place of caring, of a beloved patient's death, and the horror of being a helpless witness.

Sammy's brother and sister, robbed of time and attention for months—their mother visiting a child she couldn't mourn as dead, nor hope to laugh with again.

And his father, led to an act most people will misunderstand, an act he'll have to live with the rest of his life.

Crossing the Line to Active Euthanasia

Bioethics, you'd like to think, would be a stable field from year to year. After all, the basic ideas about moral behavior don't change that much. But the fact is, the ethical dilemmas faced by you and your doctor have changed as much in the last five years as the arsenal of pills and procedures has.

To see how fast and far we've moved, try to get hold of a surprisingly clear and frank article called "The Physician's Responsibility Toward Hopelessly Ill Patients," signed by twelve prominent physicians and printed in the prestigious *New England Journal of Medicine* in May 1989. These are not pioneers pushing the frontiers of medical ethics, but established clinicians at the center of the profession, speaking through medicine's most respected channel.

There are some surprising suggestions in the article, including the one (by ten of the twelve authors) that stated that at certain times "it is not immoral for a physician to assist in the rational suicide of a terminally ill person."

That's the one the news media picked up. Here are five others, less spectacular but just as important to us patients, from among the many in six pages of small type:

• **Artificial feeding.** "Many physicians and ethicists now agree that there is little difference between [artificial feeding and liquids] and other life-sustaining measures. They have concluded, therefore, that it is ethical to withdraw nutrition and hydration from certain dying, hopelessly ill or permanently unconscious patients."

• **Imminent death as a requirement for withdrawing support.** Courts are moving toward "the view that patients are entitled to be allowed to die, whether or not they are terminally ill or suffering"—those who are permanently unconscious, for example.

• **Doctors' reluctance.** Although more than eighty court decisions have supported or expanded patients' right to refuse treatment, there is "a large gap between what the courts now allow . . . and what physicians actually do." All too frequently, physicians are reluctant to withdraw aggressive treatment from hopelessly ill patients, despite clear legal precedent. "Physicians have a responsibility to consider timely discussions with patients about life-sustaining treatment and terminal care. Only a minority of physicians now do so consistently."

• **Educating about power.** "Medical educators need to recognize that practitioners may not sufficiently understand or value the patient's role in medical decision-making or may be unwilling to relinquish control of the decision-making process."

• **Living wills.** "Thirty-eight states now have legislation covering advance directives ('living wills'), and fifteen states

99

specifically provide that a patient's health care spokesperson, or proxy, can authorize the withholding or withdrawal of life support.'' Patients should be asked, ''on admission (to the hospital or nursing home), to indicate whether they have prepared a living will or designated a surrogate.''

Many patients and professionals will see this statement of twelve physicians as proof that the ''slippery slope'' leads only downward. Others will see the changes as the new day dawning. In between, there will be many heated discussions, as we feel our way toward a more humane and just practice of medicine.

Just remember: The best policy grows out of the widest involvement. As many patients as possible need to be active in the discussion.

Outside the ICU: A Guide to the Hardest Choices

''I know I did the wrong thing,'' he said. ''But when the doctor put the question to me, my mind just went blank.''

He wasn't the only one. As you read this, there are hundreds of relatives in waiting rooms outside intensive care units, wrestling with questions they never had to face before. Usually the questions asked by the doctor boil down to this: ''How long shall we continue fighting for the patient's life? Shall we continue the life support and other therapy? Or shall we abandon the fight and simply make the patient comfortable?''

Most people don't even know where to start when answering these questions. The mind shifts into idle, and the temptation is to hand the decision over to the nearest authority figure.

But it doesn't have to be this way. Any of us can be prepared to make a thoughtful, rational decision in a situation like this.

Thinking about the possibilities in advance—before your mind is clouded by worry and fear—will help. So will a list of questions to ask of the "physician of record" or "case manager."

Here are the questions I suggest to clients, to help them make the decision that's right for them. You may want to copy and save this list.

• **Medical questions.** When treatment is clearly futile, physicians are not required to continue giving it. Whether it's aspirin or a respirator, if it's not helping the patient get better, withdrawal may be a purely medical question. Ask the doctor:

How much chance is there that the patient can get better? How much improvement is it reasonable to expect?

How much pain is there? Is there suffering—emotional pain, despair? Is there loss of mobility?

Can the pain be fully relieved? Will the patient ever be able to move around? Communicate? Be free of pain?

Is the treatment truly therapeutic—"serving to cure or heal or preserve health," as the *New World Dictionary* puts it? How long is it likely to go on?

If the medical case is clear, the questions might stop there. But in the new medicine, there's always one more thing to try. When the question shifts from "What'll we try next?" to "Should we keep trying?" you've moved from medicine into ethics.

• **The patient's wishes.** This is the most crucial of the ethics questions. If the patient is competent, the decision is his or hers to make—whether the family agrees or not. Some questions:

Is the patient mentally competent? Able to communicate? (If the answer is no on the first one, be sure it's an opinion from a qualified specialist.)

Has the patient been fully informed of the choices, limits, and possible consequences involved?

If unable to communicate, has the patient filled out either a

Durable Power of Attorney or a Directive to Physicians ("living will")? Or did the patient ever express an opinion, orally or in a letter, about what to do?

• **External factors.** These don't have as much weight as the first two classes of questions, but may help clarify your decision.

Do the family members agree on what the patient would want? Will they support the patient in the decision?

Would any of the possible decisions put an intolerable financial burden on the relatives? Stress? Intolerable guilt?

• **Where to get help.** The best place to raise these questions is in a family conference with the key caregivers. Ask the nurses or the social worker to set it up. You can ask that your pastor, priest, or rabbi be there.

If you feel you're not being heard, ask to see the hospital's ethics committee or a clinical ethicist; their job is to help all parties sort out the alternatives, so you can make your own decision.

And carry this little list with you; it'll be a start toward making that decision your own.

Sometimes Things Go Right

Those of us who are full-time bioethicists are like cops and relief pitchers; we get called in when things go wrong. We spend much of our careers looking at trouble, and trying to help people out of it. If we aren't careful, it can get gloomy. It's easy to find refuge in a sour and cynical approach to the health care system, to the foibles of scientists and doctors and, eventually, to life in general.

There's a temptation to feel like Charlie Brown, after pitching a 13-0 losing game. Linus tells him, "Well, Charlie Brown, you win some, and you lose some."

Charlie Brown says: "That would be nice."

It's appropriate to remind ourselves that humanity does win some—that there are many times when things do go right.

A dear relative of mine, eighty-eight years old and in reasonably good health, suffered a heart attack. After a couple of days in the coronary care unit, she was alert and even able to walk a little, but exhausted and in a lot of pain. There might be another attack, or she might eventually go home in pretty good health.

And the doctor asked her children the question so many of you have been asked: If things get worse, how much should we do to save her life?

By coincidence, I was in that Rocky Mountain state that day, on a lecture tour. I had a chance to see her, and to listen to some of the family's discussion. Without any help from me, they did the right things. They faced the dilemma squarely, and they asked the right questions.

They knew what their mother wanted, and they respected her wishes. They affirmed her request to be made as comfortable as possible, but not to be resuscitated, not to be subjected to heroic treatment, if there was another attack.

She had had eighty-eight feisty, creative, and productive years. Her vision and her hearing had been diminishing; she was tired, and now there was severe pain. She was ready to rest.

Many families that I have consulted in that situation argue bitterly against the patient's right to just let go. Not surprisingly, relatives demanding that "everything be done" are often those who neglected the patient before.

Recently, I heard a man tell a nurse that his mother "had no right" to ask that intrusive treatment be stopped so she could die peacefully.

I've also seen doctors deny a patient's right to choose—to accept or deny further treatment. Such doctors, although serious and well-intentioned, often are unable to understand death as anything but professional failure.

They argue that the patient is "too depressed to make a rational decision," or that they might be sued by the survivors if they don't go into a full-court press against death.

It's usually different with the nurses. They're the ones who spend the long hours with the suffering patient, and they're usually the ones who call for a moderator—the hospital ethics committee, a pastor or rabbi, an ethicist, a social worker—when the patient's wish is being violated.

If my relative had chosen to fight fiercely to the end, I'm sure the family would have supported her in that, too. The decision, they felt, was hers to make.

In the end, no further decision was necessary. After the last daughter arrived, spent the afternoon and evening with her and tucked her into bed, she dozed off—and died in the middle of the night without waking. It was a natural part of a rich life, and it was peaceful—in part because the family, supported by the doctors and nurses, did three things right: They talked ahead of time about what to do, not waiting for a new crisis to hit. They looked realistically at the options, not avoiding hard choices. And finally, they affirmed their mother as a person when they respected the decisions she had made.

It was a good reminder to me that there are ethical wins as well as losses in the tense hush of an intensive-care unit.

PART EIGHT
CHANGING TIMES FOR DOCTORS, NURSES, AND PATIENTS

*B*y the time she'd changed into a sterile gown and was lacing up her Reeboks, she'd stopped humming the carol from the car tape-player. Her mind was on the unit, half dread and half anticipation. Rankin, the day charge nurse, greeted her with a tired grin. "Great news. Foster called in sick. There'll be just two of you ICU-certified; the other four are from the temp. registry."

She fought down resentment as Rankin went on, working through the clipboards on each patient. It hadn't been this bad before the business types took over, running the place like a factory. Six ICU-certified nurses lost in a month and not replaced. Two hundred nurses, a third of the staff, gone from the hospital in a year. Burnout, short staffs, pay freezes . . . Wryly, she flashed on the days when nurses were "angels of mercy," not budget items.

She said goodnight to Rankin and went directly to Bed 5, Emma Whittier. She felt Emma's eyes following her as she checked: IVs OK, airway clear. Chest rising and falling in rhythm with the sighing of the machine.

She kept up a cheerful chatter, but it was one-way; ALS, Lou Gehrig's disease, had long since left Emma unable to move anything but her eyes.

She held up the transparent plastic alphabet board, peering through it at Emma's eyes to see which letter the eyes focused on.

"P." Then the "L." Letter by letter, they struggled through: "P-L-E-A-S-E- L-E-T- D-I-E. P-L-E-A-S-E."

Despairing, she tried to explain that a nurse was subject to the doctor's orders, even when she felt they were wrong. She gave up halfway through, embarrassed. For a long time she just stood there, holding Emma's hand in hers, looking into those eyes.

Then she moved briskly to her other patients. Through the night hours, young Joe Walsh slept peacefully, as he had for weeks, as he might for months. Arthur Frazier tossed and moaned as she changed his dressing; she checked the orders and prepared a syringe for pain. Eye on the clock, she took a moment to massage his tight neck muscles. . . .

The shrill buzz of the alarm. Red light flashing. On Emma's monitor, a quavery, crazy line. She hit the code button and grabbed the crash cart. Harrison was already compressing Emma's chest. She put a bag over the tired gray face and began squeezing air into the lungs.

The respiratory technician loped in, followed by the emergency room doctor, in baggy greens. He grabbed the wired paddles from the cart: "Stand clear." Emma's body jerked once. Twice. A third time. Medicine into the vein to shock the heart. Again, the three powerful shocks. Ventilator on full. Then suddenly it was quiet. The resident sighed and shook his head. One by one, the team drifted away.

She began pulling the tape off Emma's body, removing the wires and tubes. Gently she pulled the lids down over the tired brown eyes. "Good night, Emma," she said. She washed the body and covered it with a light blanket.

She made the rounds of her sleeping charges once more, reported on them to her replacement, and headed for her locker, nearly an hour past quitting time. She wondered idly how long it had been since she'd had time to give a real back rub.

By the time she got home, there was light rimming the East Bay hills. Dick and the baby, still groggy from sleep, were eating breakfast. "Hi," he said. "How'd it go?"

"Oh, pretty much the usual," she said, and sat down to take off her shoes.

Medical Records: Naked to the World?

"It's not the semi-private room I object to," says the patient, hunching over beside his hospital bed. "It's the semi-private gown I don't like!"

Privacy. Highly valued, from the child who wants people to knock before entering her room to the Supreme Court, which has suggested that a right to privacy is inherent, between the lines, in the Constitution.

But in the long struggle for patients' rights, the defense of the right to privacy has turned out to be one of the toughest. Consider, for example, your medical records.

The intimate details of our medical histories, once closely guarded and inviolate, are known to an increasing number of people, in and out of the health team. It's not that people can't keep a secret any more. But the medical revolution since World War II—the same one that has given us healthier and longer lives—has made it harder to keep the confidentiality we once could count on.

Old Doc Sawbones, in the neighborhoods or small towns from which many of us came, kept our records on 3 × 5 cards in a shoe box. Our secrets were safe with him or her, to be used only for our benefit.

But two things are happening that could turn your record into a weapon that does you harm:

• The fence of privacy is full of holes and is falling down.
• Employers' health insurance costs have zoomed.

The coincidence of these two developments means that many employers, determined to bring down costs, are getting access to workers' records and using them to avoid hiring people whose health might turn bad.

A University of Illinois survey found in 1988 that half the *Fortune* 500 companies use employees' medical records routinely to make decisions about hiring, placement, promotion, and firing. That's double the number who responded that way in a survey twelve years earlier. Most of the workers affected didn't know the boss had their records. Most hadn't given permission for the records' release.

Here are some of the reasons the medical privacy that we've always taken for granted is fading fast:

• **Specialization and the proliferation of health care workers.** "Everybody has access to a patient's records today," says a neurologist friend. "The hospitals are filled with people coming and going. They all read the charts—the house staff, the nurses, the social workers, the technicians, the occupational therapists. I even see the candy-stripers flipping through the charts as they wheel people to X ray."

It's not that anybody deliberately betrays a confidence. But with so many people, there are bound to be slips. And the same expansion of personnel has hit the doctor's office.

• **Mobility.** A third of us move each year, leaving behind a trail of records and starting new ones wherever we arrive.

Think for a moment how many places must have tidbits of your medical history. Just for starters, try summer camp, grade and high schools, the military, any company you ever worked for, any doctor or hospital that ever treated you, any lab that analyzed samples, and any company from which you bought health or life insurance. It's not that any of these institutions treats your privacy casually. But sheer numbers make leaks inevitable.

And long after a record has ceased to be relevant, it can zap a career. Ask ex-Senator Tom Eagleton, who had been picked to run for vice-president until somebody found in his records that he had seen a psychiatrist years earlier.

• **Third-party payers.** He who pays the piper has a paper to fill out, whether it's a health insurance form, or Medicare or

Medicaid forms. You might not notice the fine print at the bottom when you authorize payment for removal of an ingrown toenail, but it gives the paying agency—and anybody it designates—access to your full record.

• **The computer.** It's the computer that brings all these leaks together and gives them the power to hurt you. Much of the information the insurance companies get from your records ends up in the Boston-based databank they share—well over a hundred million peoples' records. Data also pour into this facility from credit bureaus, the Defense Department, the Veterans Administration, and even Medicare and Medicaid. You can ask to see what they have on you, but you'll be refused. An employer or an insurance company can get the whole thing.

And you can be sure that the purpose is not to make you healthier, but to make sure they don't hire or insure a "clunker." That's the trade nickname for somebody they'd rather not insure. If you're a clunker, it could be bad news for you personally.

But the harm may be to all of us. Dr. Alan Westin, author of "Privacy and Freedom," says that the amassing of so much personal information, "in a way we sometimes only dimly grasp, is one of the great changes in our society."

Eye Doc Made Him See Red

In Lake Worth, Florida, a businessman struck a blow for patients everywhere. William Ennis had sent his eye doctor a bill for $90 because the doctor was a full hour late for an appointment. Ennis figured his own time was worth about that much.

When his doctor ignored the bill, Ennis sent several more notices. Then he sued.

The doctor said he was flabbergasted—that he'd had five

emergencies that morning and couldn't possibly have been on time. Ennis finally offered to drop the matter if the physician would make a $90 donation to the Lions Club's eye fund. We all won a minor victory when the doctor agreed to make the contribution.

Now, my own eye doctor is a warm and lovable man. He cares deeply about his patients, and I've seen his eyes mist over when he was describing a patient who might lose her vision. I'm told he is the best in the area in his specialized field. The nurses and technicians on his staff like working for him, and enjoy a level of mutual respect that is impossible with some M.D.s.

If you have the kind of eye trouble he specializes in, you'd be lucky to have him working on you. Just don't expect him ever to be on time. Last time I was there, I waited an hour for the drops to dilate my pupils, and then another thirty-five minutes past the appointment time—less than usual—before being called in to the examining room. But then I sat there another thirty-five minutes while he took a phone call (non-medical), made a phone call (non-medical), discussed with a nurse the previous patient's pleasant personality, and, finally, discussed with a nurse various remedies for his dog's loneliness. The eye exam itself, when he got around to it, took fifteen minutes.

When he was done, I was fuming. Altogether, I had spent two hours, plus travel, for a fifteen-minute exam. Even worse was the fact that my wife, Virginia, had driven me there because of what the drops do to my eyes; she also had wasted two hours.

For me, that kind of thing is not a disaster; it's just inconvenient and a destruction of a limited resource—time. But what about people who have a difficult time getting off work, and lose pay for every hour they miss? Or single parents who have to find child care? Or people waiting in severe pain?

The number of doctors who do this to their patients is much

less than it used to be, but it still happens. Why? Here are some of the theories proposed by a nonscientific panel of friends:

• **Emergencies.** This can happen to any doctor. But what about the ones who are always late?

• **Overscheduling.** Maybe the doctor has too many patients and just can't keep up. If this is really the case, respect for patients and good medical care call for cutting back.

• **Disorganization.** My other doctor also carries a heavy case load, but I always get in within two minutes of the appointed time. Does he know more about organization and discipline?

• **Impaired doctor:** Maybe the physician is one of those whose performance is impaired by drug or alcohol abuse.

• **Overconsideration:** The doctor cares so much that he or she spends extra time with each patient. But where's the concern for the patient out in the waiting room, reading a 1984 *Reader's Digest*?

• **Insecurity:** Maybe, one friend suggests, it confirms a physician's sense of importance to see so many people willing to wait and wait.

• **Behind the times:** This is my theory: A doctor who consistently sees patients late is a victim of the old belief that a physician's time is more valuable than any other person's. It's a relic of the days when the doctor was priest, scientist, healer, and magician all wrapped into one. The attitude is ethically unacceptable, because it dehumanizes the patient. And it is bound to damage the doctor-patient relationship.

So what should one do? Sending a bill or suing isn't for everybody. But you can confront the doctor. Explain the inconvenience—something that may not have occurred to him or her. Point out, politely but firmly, that your time is also valuable—and that such thoughtlessness would be unacceptable in, say, a social setting.

And if you're too chicken to do that, there's one other measure to take: Write a chapter in a book about it.

What It Means When You Hurt

A prominent group of doctors says there's no reason a dying patient should have to suffer pain, no matter how bad the medical condition. But that doesn't guarantee that your own doctor will practice medicine that way. Doctors' attitudes toward relieving pain reflect our society's—and have to do more with ancestry and religion, with values and emotions than with modern medicine.

Many doctors will still prescribe, every four hours, only enough pain reliever to last two or three hours. Many patients suffer such agony that tears and sweat roll down their cheeks together, but won't ask for, or can't get, relief. It's not that science doesn't know how to relieve pain. It's that many doctors are not sure they want to.

The landmark article on "The Physician's Responsibility Toward Hopelessly Ill Patients," written by twelve physicians at ten major medical centers, puts this horrifying truth in the flat, objective language of science: "One of the most pervasive causes of anxiety among patients . . . is the perception that physicians' efforts toward the relief of pain are sadly deficient. . . . People fear that needless suffering will be allowed to occur as patients are dying. To a large extent, we believe such fears are justified."

Here are a few of the reasons we fight pain half-heartedly:

• **Religion.** In her provocative 1978 book, *The Politics of Pain*, Helen Neal summed up the work of several researchers when she said, "What we may think is an automatic response to pain and suffering most likely has been conditioned in us by the religious beliefs of our ancestors."

The historic Jewish attitude, for example, is that there is no virtue in suffering; it is a condition to be avoided, not sought. Many Christians, on the other hand, spiritualize pain, interpreting it as sent by God—to punish us for our individual and corporate sins, to test our faith, or to challenge us to spiritual growth. There is, of course, a vast difference between using pain as an occasion to grow in character, and believing that God would deliberately cause us to suffer so that we might grow.

• **Frustration with the chronic.** Medical training is aimed at acute situations and quick solutions; conditions that go on and on are frustrating and boring for the physician.

• **Only a symptom.** Since pain is often a warning of some serious condition, it's easy to dismiss the pain part as unimportant and concentrate only on the underlying cause.

• **Drug phobia.** Decades of various ''wars'' on street drugs have clouded our minds about pain killers. A prominent pharmacologist, dean of a medical school, once told me he would not use narcotics to ease the pain of a cancer patient, just days from death, if he felt the patient might become addicted. This same phobia forbids U.S. doctors the use of heroin, a more effective (and less depressive) pain killer than morphine.

• **Machismo.** If you can't take a little pain, you're not a man.

• **Sexism.** A macho society has told us that a woman's pain is, likely as not, ''all in her head.'' Research shows a higher percentage of doctors are more likely to consider pain as irrelevant if the patient is a woman.

In response to all this, the authors of the journal article mentioned above are clear and firm:

''The hopelessly ill patient must have whatever is necessary to control pain. Under no circumstances should medication be 'rationed.' '' For, ''To allow a patient to experience unbearable pain or suffering is unethical medical practice.''

Whose Doctors Are They, Anyway?

Charlie Krueger, a lineman for the San Francisco '49ers for sixteen years, raised questions about the doctor-patient relationship by going to court over it. Krueger sued the team and its doctors in 1981 for letting him play for nearly ten of those years with an injured left knee.

The team doctors never told him, the lawsuit said, that playing on the knee could cripple him permanently. In fact, Krueger said, they injected him with pain-killers and steroids, and he was directed to keep on playing.

Today Krueger, after unsuccessful surgery, "cannot stand for prolonged periods and cannot run. He is unable to walk on stairs without severe pain. His condition is degenerative and irreversible."

Those are the words of a California state Court of Appeals, which ruled that the team had "consciously failed to make full, meaningful disclosure to him respecting the magnitude of the risk he took in continuing to play."

In a similar suit ten years earlier, Bill Enyart, a middle linebacker for the (then) Oakland Raiders, charged the Raiders' physicians with malpractice, saying they induced him to play the last half of an exhibition game on a severely injured knee. He was awarded more than $400,000.

The Hippocratic oath says, "The health and life of my patient will be my first consideration." When we walk into a doctor's office, we believe that's the unspoken agreement. And most of the time, that trust is well-placed.

But it's not a bad idea to remind ourselves that there are situations in which the patient comes in a distant second. These may not be as dramatic as the scene in the Raiders' locker room, with the team behind in the last quarter, but they are very real.

Think, for example, about the doctor paid by an insurance

company to examine you. His or her "first consideration" is not your health; it's the company's. The purpose of the exam is to keep bad risks off the rolls, and the doctor's aim is to discover anything at all that might disqualify you. In this situation, what you trustingly reveal is not protected by the ideal of confidentiality, and could actually be used against you. It's all up-front, legal and, in many people's eyes, ethically acceptable. Just don't make the mistake of thinking that this is the standard doctor-patient encounter.

An extreme example of corporate loyalty was revealed recently: Some insurance-company doctors were sending applicants' blood samples, without their knowledge, through one extra test—for the AIDS virus. These doctors not only violated the professional obligation of getting informed consent, but were breaking a California state law against involuntary HIV testing, and another law forbidding insurance companies to disqualify HIV carriers.

There's another situation in which a doctor, no matter how well-intentioned, can end up breaching the patient's trust and making the patient's interests secondary: medical research. As the public, we've been so well exposed to the value of research, the great stories of "breakthroughs" made possible by experimentation on human subjects, that we forget to ask questions about the fate of those subjects.

In the late nineteenth century, when the form of ethical evaluation called Utilitarianism was the rage, results were what counted. The experimental subject's suffering was for the "greater good"—a cure, perhaps, for thousands yet unborn. This idea is increasingly under fire, even in the current federal regulations for human research. But it lives on, and is clearly another exception to the ideal of putting the patient's life and health first.

Those artificial-heart patients, existing in a semicoma, hitched permanently to 300-pound carts, had believed they were being treated for their own good—that therapy was the doctors' goal, that this would be a "cure" for their dying condition. Maybe their doctors believed this too. But in the long run, after their suffering had ended, hindsight made it clear that the only justification for putting them through all this was the knowledge gained, knowledge that might help others. That's okay if Barney Clark and the others knew from the start that they were guinea pigs, not patients—and that their doctors' primary concern was knowledge for others, not therapy for them.

Some of the situations described here pose no real ethical problem for the physician, and some are real dilemmas. But for us patients, there's no dilemma; if our doctor is working on somebody else's agenda, we should be made aware of it, and be able to decide whether we want to continue the relationship.

Can Your Doctor Fire You?

You know you have a right to fire your doctor. But when does the doctor have a right to fire you?

The question came up when a California judge ordered a doctor to give thirty-eight-year-old Jeanie Joshua one more week of kidney dialysis. But after that, the judge said, she'd have to look elsewhere.

Joshua says she has no place else to go. Every other dialysis center within reach has turned her down, she says—eleven doctors in all. No, it's not that Joshua doesn't have health insurance. And it isn't that she doesn't need the "kidney machine" treatment; without it, she'll die, painfully, in a couple of weeks.

The thing that makes her the Flying Dutchman of California health care, wandering the coast from clinic to clinic, is this: A couple of years ago, she sued a doctor. In a suit that hasn't yet been settled, she charged a doctor with using impure water in the dialysis machine.

There's more: Joshua's physician told a newspaper he was dropping her as a patient because she was "too aggressive" in directing her own medical treatment. Joshua describes herself as an "assertive" patient, who sometimes refuses treatment or tests she doesn't agree with.

I've often heard doctors gossiping about patients who "don't want to follow orders," who "think they know more than I do about medicine," or who are "malpractice types." It's easy to sympathize with their attitude. Doctors put up with an unusual amount of stress. Most work long, hard hours. The responsibility can be crushing. Who needs an ungrateful patient, or one who doesn't respect your expertise?

The right to choose your own patients, after all, is the foundation of American medical practice. Its (alleged) absence is one of the arguments most often made against national health programs. In Joshua's case, her doctor's lawyer says, "It's well-established law that a physician may select which patients he cares for."

But wait a second. Like so much that physicians "know" about non-medical topics, that's only half the story. Jeanie Joshua is entitled to certain minimum health care, and she doesn't give that up when she exercises other rights, like suing or speaking up.

The doctor, meanwhile, has a right to withdraw from the case, but, according to the American Medical Association, has a clear responsibility to see that the patient finds another doctor. That's because we're not selling pickles here; we're selling life and death.

The ACLU's paperback, *The Rights of Doctors, Nurses and Allied Health Professionals*—one of an excellent series that includes books on the rights of hospital patients and of the terminally ill—says that once a doctor has taken on a patient, their relationship continues until:

• It is revoked by the consent of both.
• It is revoked by the patient.
• The doctor's services are no longer necessary.
• The doctor withdraws from the case after reasonable notice to the patient.

In other words, a patient can be fired for "almost any reason so long as it is done at a point that does not jeopardize the patient's health, and ample time and notice and referral suggestions are given so that the patient can find another qualified provider."

That's a big "if." In the case of Jeanie Joshua, we can sympathize with a physician who fears she might file another malpractice suit, and maybe even understand his difficulty in learning to deal with new-style "uppity" patients. But is that enough reason to cut her off from the only treatment that stands between her and certain death?

PART NINE
PATIENTS' RIGHTS, PATIENTS' RITES

When Hector Rodas, forty-three, paralyzed from the neck down, told the doctors in a Colorado hospital he wanted to die, he had to have the help of a therapist with a letter board. But paralyzed as he was, he was lending a hand to you, me, and everyone else who is in a doctor's care once in a while.

Blinking to signal the correct letter as the therapist's pointer moved across the board, Rodas said, in one of his early messages: "Call civil rights, don't feed, I don't want food. Against." The doctors understood the message, but they refused to remove the feeding tube that ran through his nose into his stomach.

"You're too young," they said. "You have many good years ahead."

"You're too distraught to think clearly," they said. "There may be hope of regaining movement."

The hospital administration agreed. "You're asking the staff to assist in a suicide," they said. "You're clinically depressed, and thus incompetent to decide."

Rodas's response, laboriously worked out with the help of the therapist: "I am capable of making my own decisions, please help me. Don't put words in my mouth."

The hospital and doctors got a temporary court order continuing the feeding. Months later, after hearings, Judge Charles Buss ruled in Rodas's favor. The thirty-eight-page opinion drew on higher-court rulings in a dozen other states, but to a lay person, these paragraphs sum it up:

"The court finds unconvincing the opinions of these very well-meaning, highly trained, and professional [doctors and administrators] as to the issue of Mr. Rodas's capacity, because their professional opinions were so clearly influenced by their personal opinion of the rightness and wrongness in his decision. . . .

"To allow others to decide what is in his best interests would be to disregard the clearly established legal and medical ethic that a competent adult is allowed to refuse medical treatment."

The judge was talking about an ideal important to every one of us patients: "informed consent."

Informed consent, you see, is as much about consent as it is about informing. Many doctors and more patients don't realize that. When a national sample of doctors was asked, "What does the term 'informed' consent mean to you?" 59 percent mentioned "generally informing the patient," but only 26 percent mentioned "the patient giving permission for treatment."

Neither the good intentions nor the competence of physicians is in question here. We usually can assume that both are present. But the attitudes of many doctors and patients are leftovers from more paternalistic days, when professionals advised an uneducated public on all areas of life—not just the ones they were trained for. Look how easily Robert Young could move from "Father Knows Best" to "Marcus Welby, M.D." without even changing expression.

Judge Buss was reminding us what law and ethics have been saying for years—and what, through ignorance, have been among the most-violated rules in medicine: Except in emergencies when you're unable to communicate, a physician must have your informed consent before treating you for anything. This is true whether the treatment is a life-support system or a cast on a broken leg. It's true for pain pills, life-extending chemotherapy, or a radical mastectomy.

What's more, *consent* means any of these:

• The right to consent to the treatment.

• The right to refuse the treatment, no matter what the consequences.

• The right to withdraw consent already given.

And these rights apply if either the patient is conscious and competent or is represented by someone who knows what the patient would want.

A friend of mine who had attended a workshop on these matters and had discussed them with her husband was called to his bedside in the intensive care unit at 2 A.M. He was sinking fast.

She saw a big machine nearby: "What's that?"

"It's a ventilator," she was told. "We'll hook it up if he stops breathing."

"No, you won't," she said.

And they didn't.

Women Get in a Word About Bodies

Why all the fuss about "a superficial, easily disposable appendage?" the male surgeon wanted to know. He could understand why his patient was upset about having cancer, but why should she react so strongly to losing a breast?

Author Mary Spetter ran into the same attitude when she began thinking about plastic surgery to rebuild a breast lost in a mastectomy.

"Women don't need it," one surgeon (male) told her.

"Aren't you happy with your marriage? Is something wrong with your job?" another asked.

A surgeon told a reporter: "Breast reconstruction is only for women with strong self-image problems."

Spetter says U.S. doctors' typical stance toward mastectomy at that time—in 1977—was, "Your life has been saved; what more could you want? The woman who meekly replied, 'My breast,' or who reacted with prolonged tears or depression was at the least considered unappreciative and vain, and at worst possibly neurotic.''

Well, some of these attitudes changed when then-First Lady Nancy Reagan underwent surgery, and it's a safe guess that the President's wife was not exposed to such unabashed paternalism and sexism. Just as important, many of the 100,000 or so women who get breast cancer this year won't face it either.

In the last thirteen years, the medical environment has changed drastically from the one Spetter describes in her book, *A Woman's Choice*. It's a change worth thinking about, and not just for women; it's a model of the change taking place in all of health care. And it's a vivid reminder of how much our self-image is tied to our body. Ethics and medicine are intertwined, in the kind of classic bioethics questions both sexes face.

Here are some of the important changes in recent years:

• **New options for treatment.** Although British surgeons had had good results in the 1940s with simple mastectomy followed by radiation, most U.S. surgeons clung to the ninety-year tradition of "radical" mastectomy—removing also the lymph nodes in the armpit and muscles of the chest.

It wasn't until 1979 that an international conference convened by the National Institutes of Health led to a recommendation that the "radical" be abandoned; the experts said other forms were less mutilating and had fewer complications. There are still doctors who argue that the radical mastectomy is the only way to be sure of getting all the cancer. But under the right conditions, women can choose alternatives like the modified radical, the partial mastectomy, and the lumpectomy, with equal odds for survival.

• **Biopsy separate from the surgery.** Since the nineteenth century, it has been the practice to examine a possibly cancerous breast lump in the operating room, with the patient asleep under anesthesia. If the lab reports that the tissue is malignant, the surgeons proceed with a mastectomy.

But the same NIH panel in 1979 recommended a two-step procedure in most cases. The procedure, already in wide use in Europe, was simply common sense: Do the biopsy first, usually with a local anesthetic, and schedule follow-up treatment or surgery later. This way is cheaper, since you don't need a fully equipped operating room for the biopsy. It is safer because the lab pathologist has time for a more thorough look at the tumor. It also allows the patient to make arrangements for the time of hospitalization and recuperation.

Most important, it protected the patient's right to make an informed decision. While some women still prefer to trust the surgeon to make the decision for them while they sleep, most seem to agree with Shirley Temple Black, who wrote after her mastectomy: "I find intellectually distasteful the prospect of waking up and finding that someone else had made a decision and taken an action in which I, lying quite inert on the operating table, had no voice. . . . If my breast was going to be removed, I needed to be in on that decision. I wanted to take one step at a time."

• **The right to informed consent.** These changes coincided with growing recognition that patients had a right to know what their medical choices were, and to accept or reject them. Better education, the women's movement, and consumerism all contributed to the change in attitudes. And psychologists have found that women who feel they have no choice do not cope as well as those who are informed of the options.

• **Honesty about cancer.** As recently as the 1960s, most doctors wouldn't tell patients they had cancer. The AMA recommended families be told instead. Even among themselves, health professionals spoke of "the patient with 'C,' " avoiding the awful word. And newspaper obituaries always referred to it as "a lingering illness." Such mendacity, no matter how well-intentioned, had the effect of denying the patient any choice.

• **Breast reconstruction.** Anybody sensitive to the importance of self-image and aware of society's attitudes toward the breast—from motherhood to sexuality—won't question the motives of those who seek this increasingly expert procedure.

• **Education of the medical male doctor.** Men are capable of learning, despite occasional evidence to the contrary. Paternalism is on the way out. One sign: Some health insurance plans that for years had covered plastic implants for penises but not breast reconstruction now cover both.

It's interesting that Nancy Reagan, with all the new possibilities, chose the one-step biopsy and surgery, and had a radical mastectomy.

But the decision was hers.

That's the important thing.

Making Sure the Decision Is Yours

Years ago, people were terrified about going to a hospital because the odds weren't very good that they would come out alive. Ironically, a major reason many people fear the hospital today is just the opposite: the belief they might not be allowed to die.

Most of us fear, with some reason, a life in limbo, with life-support technology indefinitely postponing our natural process of dying. Given this widespread worry, I'm always surprised by how few people know about the Durable Power of Attorney (DPA) for health care.

The DPA is a simple way of naming someone you trust as your agent, or surrogate, to make health care decisions on your behalf if you ever become unable to make your own. It's available in most states. You don't need a lawyer or a notary to make one out—just two witnesses, and the permission of the decision-maker you name. It's a good idea to name a couple of alternates, and to leave copies with your doctor, lawyer, pastor or rabbi, and members of your family.

In case you're confused between the DPA and the "living will," here are some of the differences:

• **Legal status.** The living will lets you express your wish not to be given extraordinary treatment, but relies on moral, not legal, persuasion to get the doctor to comply.

The DPA is a legal document giving your surrogate the same decision-making power you would have had if you were conscious—greater than that of the doctor, family members, or anyone else.

• **Options.** The living will usually is useful only if you want treatment withheld.

With the DPA, you can also choose the opposite—everything the doctor considers medically appropriate. Or you can make a distinction, for example, between withdrawal of life support and withdrawal of food and water.

• **Protecting the doctors.** The living will doesn't protect doctors from legal trouble that might result from following your wishes; the DPA does, and thus is more likely to be followed.

• **Flexibility.** This is the biggest difference. You can't anticipate every possible situation, so a written document like the living will often won't fit the specific crisis when it occurs.

The DPA provides a living witness on the scene, one who

knows you well and can make the best guess about what you might do in such a situation.

You can pick just about any adult to be your surrogate. It makes sense, of course, to choose somebody who knows your mind. My own surrogate is my wife, Virginia; my alternate is a registered nurse who also knows my feelings about life and death. While his or her decisions will generally be legally binding on the health care team, there are some things your surrogate usually won't be allowed to agree to: commitment to a mental health facility, electroshock or other convulsive treatment, psychosurgery, sterilization, or abortion. If your surrogate decides treatment should be withdrawn, the doctor will make every effort to communicate with you; if by some miracle that happens and you disagree with the decision, your own decision carries, of course.

The DPA is a way of ensuring that your autonomy and right to decision-making are respected, even in the comatose last stages of life. It can stave off many regrets, and save your family much agony. So, in hopes of nudging a few people into action, here are answers to some of the questions that come up. The specifics vary from state to state, but these answers are generally true:

• Do I need a lawyer for this? No. The DPA is in plain English and can be witnessed by two acquaintances or one notary public.

• Can I be denied health insurance if I don't sign a DPA? Or refused admission to a hospital? Since your surrogate might be able to prevent a long and pointless extension of your dying, insurers or hospitals might gain from requiring every client to fill one out. But this is specifically forbidden under most states' laws.

• What if my family disagrees with my surrogate? Your surrogate prevails, because under the law he or she is a stand-in for you. This is especially important these days in the life-and-death decisions of AIDS cases, where a dying person's long-term partner may be excluded from decisions, or even from the hospital room, because society doesn't recognize the relationship.

If there isn't a DPA, a patient's wishes could be ignored by family members who have been estranged or out of touch, but are heard by hospital personnel. The DPA gives legal decision-making power to the person you want to speak for you.

• I know my agent can refuse treatment for me, but what if I want all the treatment I can get? Then just tell your agent that's what you'll want. The DPA, unlike the Directive to Physicians, the so-called "living will," allows either choice.

• Can I choose witnesses from among my relatives or heirs? One of the two witnesses must be a person who is not related to you and doesn't stand to inherit anything from you.

• How do I know my agent will make the decision I want? You make sure of this by (1) choosing somebody who knows you well and whom you trust, (2) talking at length with her or him about your wishes, and (3) writing specific preferences, if you wish, in the DPA.

• What if I've named my spouse as agent, and we get divorced? Don't worry; the designation of your spouse is automatically revoked by divorce.

• What if I change my mind and want to call the whole thing off? You can revoke the DPA, making it null and void, as the lawyers say, merely by telling the doctor or nurse.

• Is one copy enough? Legally, yes. But if you're wise, you'll make photocopies to leave with your surrogate and the alternates, with other family members, your pastor or rabbi, your doctors, and your lawyer. Giving copies to anyone who might be around at the crucial time also gives you a chance to discuss your wishes with the person getting the copy.

• Is all this really necessary? Can't I just trust my relatives or my doctor to do the right thing? (1) Yes. (2) No. Family members disagree with one another. Doctors, no matter how well-intentioned, may substitute their wishes for yours. The DPA is your best insurance that you are the one, in the long run, making decisions about your own life and death.

Drug Abuse of a Different Sort

You've seen her—on TV or in the movies, if not in the back room of some nursing home.

Her head jerks forward and her tongue pops out and down, almost touching her chin. And then she does it again. And again. And again and again.

She fits the picture we kids used to have of the "crazy people" inside as we crept cautiously past the state hospital in my home town. But the pain in those eyes, trapped in that jerking head, tells you she is only too well aware of her condition.

The doctors have a term for this spastic, Parkinson-like jerking, this ghastly lashing-out of the tongue. It's called tardive dyskinesia. What the doctors don't have is a cure for it.

The irony is that the condition was caused by a drug given her not to make her well but to keep her quiet. There weren't enough people on the staff to watch everybody, and she was too frail to be allowed to move about on her own.

"Chemical restraints" is what they called this use of the powerful mood-altering drugs to keep perfectly sane people under control, to keep the old folks from crawling out of bed and hurting themselves. "Far more humane," the staff said, "than leather straps on the wrists and across the chest."

How were they to know, in the mid-1970s, that a long time on a psychoactive drug could cause irreversible tardive dyskinesia? Or an incessant rash? Or pneumonia? Or depression? Or loss of such indefinables as dignity, awareness, or quality of life?

She was never asked whether she wanted the drug. If she had been mentally ill, informed-consent laws would have required that she or her next of kin give permission. But in a nursing home, at that time, she had no clearly spelled-out rights.

Back in 1976, the federal government surveyed nursing homes and found "chemical restraints" used on an alarming percentage of elderly patients. Warnings went out. Articles and editorials appeared in the medical journals. Over the years, researchers documented the dangerous side effects of the psychoactive drugs when misused. Too late to help the woman with tardive dyskinesia and her suffering brothers and sisters, but certainly in time to help others. And there's the real tragedy. Because not one thing has changed.

In 1988 and 1989, two national studies showed that misuse and overuse of "chemical restraints" is as common as ever. To be exact, Dr. Jerry Avorn of Harvard found that "30 percent of nursing home residents get long-acting benzodiazepines strong enough to sedate them or make them prone to falling."

We could blame the nursing homes, a third of whom, according to a recent federal study, don't bother to get a doctor's written order for such prescriptions.

We could blame the nursing home operators, many of whom see their establishments only as investments, and squeeze staffing until the patients bleed.

We could blame the doctors, as Dr. Avorn does, who "prescribed the wrong drug in the wrong dose, or prescribed it when none was needed." The basic ethics question—informed consent by the patient for such medication—doesn't even come up.

We could blame nurses who get callous in the face of such suffering.

We could blame the pharmaceutical industry for not following up on this misuse.

But those are the wrong places to put blame for the woman with the grotesque facial contortions. As long as health care is a business, answerable more to stockholders than to the sick, it will be natural for some entrepreneurs to emphasize profit, cost-cutting, the convenience of overworked staffs, and warehousing, not care. And the chemical restrainers will find a way to continue, no matter what the consequences to their frail patients.

Winning the Battle with the Machines

The spaceship crew in *2001* finally put Hal, the uppity computer, back in his box. In the final minutes of *War Games,* the kid outsmarted the hard drive that threatened to nuke the world.

And back here in the real world, we may at last be winning the battle of the machines that took over medicine. It was a close call. Like the microwave and the automatic teller machine, the machinery of medical technology can do great good, and we welcomed its amazing benefits. Most of us know people whose lives have been saved by the respirator, intravenous feeding, the artificial kidney, the pacemaker, or the defibrilator.

As these great devices were being developed, doctors were also becoming much more aggressive against illness. Powerful new drugs and the new machinery encouraged them to intervene in situations that before World War II would have called just for keeping the patient comfortable. Lives were saved; loved ones lived on.

But somewhere during this time we began letting the machines take over. Without fanfare, their role just naturally expanded— from saving lives that might have been lost to arbitrarily extending lives that might mercifully have been over. We began making decisions in which the machine, not the patient's needs and wishes, was the major factor. More often than not, the new machines were kept pumping and slushing away even after it stopped making sense from the patient's point of view.

The mystique of the machine, the godlike aura of the scientific gadget, had fogged the minds of health care professionals. A doctor might not give a second thought to discontinuing a drug that wasn't doing any good, but would say, ''I can't disconnect the ventilator, even though there is no hope, because it would be immoral.''

In a distortion of real science, we were caught up in a phony worship of technology, with these as its commandments:

• If we have the ability to do something, we always should do it. (''Since we know how to provide total nutrition through IV fluids, not to do so is murder by starvation.'')

• The decision to begin mechanical life support is radically different from the decision to withdraw it. (''Intervening in the natural course of a fatal illness is not 'playing God,' but withdrawing the artificial interference is.'')

• The one who alone understands the mysteries of the machine is the one who should make decisions about its use. (''In my clinical judgment, it would be immoral to do this, no matter what the family says.'')

Under the reign of the machine, doctors were afraid they'd be sued for malpractice if they didn't use every pill and gadget they had to win a few more hours of life. Patients and families, awed by what science has wrought, hesitated to question the rightness of the technological full-court press.

One day somebody counted up. There were, on any given day, 10,000 to 25,000 such hostages to technology, suspended between life and death, in the hospitals of the United States.

But already the course of the war with the machines was turning. Encouraged by the consumers' and women's movements, patients were asking common-sense questions about their care. Thoughtful physicians and nurses were realizing that doing one's utmost was sometimes the cruelest kind of medicine. The new discipline of bioethics was changing the nature of discussion in medical schools. And the courts were beginning to drive the machines back into their proper place.

The first big right-to-die decision was in 1976, when the New Jersey Supreme Court said Karen Ann Quinlan's parents had the right to decide whether to keep their irreversibly comatose daughter on a respirator. Other decisions followed so swiftly that within five years the debate centered not on artificial breathing, but on an even more emotional issue: artificial feeding.

In 1981 murder charges were filed against two L.A. doctors who removed, at the family's request, intravenous feeding tubes from a patient in a persistent vegetative state. Three successive courts threw out the charges.

By the end of 1987, six appeals courts in four states had said (1) high-technology feeding is a medical procedure, not a basic support function, and (2) the decision about starting or stopping it is the age-old decision about refusing treatment, and belongs to the patient, if competent. If not, then to relatives or a designated surrogate.

Since then, according to Paul Armstrong, Karen Ann Quinlan's lawyer, there have been so many right-do-die decisions that the emphasis now is not on establishing rights, but on creation ''nationwide of tort remedies for failure to honor those wishes.''

There are still skirmishes in the intensive-care units. But the outcome is inevitable. The life-extending machines, like Hal, are being put in their place as servants, not masters, of humankind.

PART TEN
GETTING HEALTH CARE
BACK ON TRACK

———————————

Who lives and who dies, in this day of high-tech, hard-choice medicine? Is there any sense, any pattern to the choices?

Look at these four news stories—all from the national news services in the same week—and see what your conclusion would be:

■　■　■

WASHINGTON, D.C.—A federal judge has refused to order Virginia's Medicaid system to pay for a liver transplant needed to save the life of four-year-old Michelle Todd.

U.S. District Judge Albert V. Bryan, Jr., in denying the motion, said Michelle's hardship had to be weighed against the finite resources of the state and the competing interests of other transplant candidates. "How can they sentence a baby to death?" said her distraught father, twenty-six-year-old Michael Todd, after the decision.

About forty of the fifty states authorize Medicaid payments for liver transplants. Children's Hospital of Pittsburgh will not perform the surgery without an advance payment of $162,000.

The Todds' attorneys said they will appeal. In addition, a fundraising drive to pay for Michelle's operation was started by the county treasurer.

■　■　■

CHICAGO—A federal judge has ordered the state to pay for bone marrow transplants for a six-year-old cancer victim. The state had balked at paying for the procedure for Crystal Shannon of Chicago Ridge because it considers such treatment experimental.

But in his order, U.S. District Judge Paul Plunkett cited affidavits from doctors that called the bone-marrow transplant Crystal's best chance for survival.

The state became involved in the case because Crystal's family receives public medical assistance and sought to have the Department of Public Aid pay for the cancer treatment.

Crystal will enter a Chicago hospital early next week. Doctors say there is a 25 to 40 percent chance of success.

■ ■ ■

MIAMI—At a news conference Maria DeSillers thanked all those who helped her raise an estimated $400,000 to save the life of her seven-year-old son, Ronnie.

Ronnie is to fly Tuesday to Pittsburgh, to be evaluated for a liver transplant. Doctors estimate he has about six months to live without it.

DeSillers, an advertising consultant, said she is trying to elicit public attention and sympathy for her son. Among the contributions for Ronnie were $200,000 from a millionaire and $1,000 from President Reagan.

"Every successful case I've heard of has had a lot of media coverage," she said. "Others have fallen between the cracks [and the children have died]. . . . I don't want Ronnie to be a case that falls through the cracks."

■ ■ ■

CHICAGO—Eight-month-old Meghann LaRocco, who has received four liver transplants, could be on her way home from the hospital within three weeks, her doctor says.

She can go home from the University of Chicago's Wyler Children's Hospital whenever she is weaned off the respirator that has helped her breathe since the third transplant, said Dr. Peter Whitington.

Her body rejected the first liver, transplanted in November. The second and third livers, transplanted two days apart in December, sustained her until a better match could be found.

■ ■ ■

What is the key to life here? Is it having a mother who's an advertising consultant? Living in the right state? Being able to afford the best lawyer? Being rich enough to pay for health care, poor enough to get public assistance, but not anywhere in between? Putting out enough cans in delicatessens and groceries, with a slot on top for spare change?

Since as a nation we seem willing to spend only a certain finite amount for health care, each highly expensive operation, including transplants, uses money that isn't available for less dramatized procedures. Is there any way to make the system more just? How would you go about it?

A Touch of Reality on the Tube

When you're sick, just call the limousine, right? Ride in style out to Walter Reed Army Hospital, where they usher you to a spacious suite. You won't have to leave the suite for tests and X rays; the technicians and their machines will come to you. So will the best doctors in the country; if they aren't already in the building, the Air Force will fly them to Bethesda in some general's jet.

Top-of-the-line care. And of course no bills to pay! So what's all this about inadequate health care? Are those agitators still trying to ruin the best medical system in the world?

■ ■ ■

Have we become the nation of the overdog? We give lip service to the downtrodden, but our hearts are really with the treaders, who not only set health care policy but define the image of it we carry around in our heads. Consider the following:

• Members of Congress, a cabinet and a president who haven't stood in line in a clinic or paid a doctor bill in years.

• Physicians, whose average income is now around $130,000, and whose own doctor bills are voided as "professional courtesy."

• A new generation of hip young executives, truly masters of business administration, fighting to keep their institutions in good health, regardless of what happens to the patients passing through.

We let the news media glibly reassure us that Britain's National Health Service is a disaster—that people have to stand in long lines, or wait weeks for an appointment. Meanwhile, we take justifiable pride—and our picture of U.S. health care—in the glistening operating rooms where teams of green-gowned geniuses use the newest machines and techniques to outwit the threat of death. There are statistics that give a different picture, of course. But statistics are pretty bloodless, pretty dull, and do little to change a picture we are determined to see.

■ ■ ■

But there's a TV documentary that made the rounds on the public channels that makes the truth so vivid that even the most determined denial is hard to maintain. It is called "Who Lives, Who Dies?" and it is a strong dose of reality from the first moment—when you hear James Earl Jones (Darth Vader in the

Star Wars) say while a series of close-ups appears on the screen:

"One of six Americans has no health insurance. As a result, this woman lost her baby. This man almost died of a brain hemorrhage. And this infant will be severely retarded.

"At the same time as we deny these people basic medical care, this former alcoholic will receive a $200,000 liver transplant. This terminal patient will remain on life support machines against her will. And this permanently comatose man will be kept alive indefinitely."

Decisions about how we will spend our health care funds, the show goes on to say, are actually decisions about who will live and who will die. We are rationing health care, sometimes by design and sometimes by default.

"The most pervasive form of rationing is denial of health care to the poor. Thirty-seven million people have no health insurance—ten million more than a decade ago."

The camera shows indigent people waiting at a county hospital, the only place left for those with no money. A pregnant woman tells us it takes five to six hours of waiting on each visit, and a hospital employee says delay has become a new way of rationing: "We have to give some people appointments six months away; there's no way they're going to keep an appointment like that."

And the Darth Vader voice points out that demand at the hospital grows while the funds across the country dwindle.

"In a decade, 800,000 women have been cut off from Medicaid. In that time, Medicaid has gone from covering 65% of the poor to 39%."

The truth about U.S. health care is not the limousine and the suite, or even the gleaming operating room. It is a shabby hall filled with waiting women, 40,000 of whom will lose their babies this year because prenatal care is too expensive, or too far away.

It's a hospital closing its pedriatric clinic because the state has cut its budget. It's a woman with a growth in her neck waiting six weeks to find out whether it's cancerous. It is 37 million people, half of them employed, who have no health care insurance at all. The brutal truth is that the "best medical system in the world" has the worst infant and maternal mortality rate of any industrialized nation.

The truth, hidden from us by various vested interests and our own determined denial, is that the United States is one of only two developed nations in the world without some form of national health coverage—some assurance that even the poorest have access to minimum, basic care. The other such country, our partner in shame, is South Africa.

Why We're Getting Sick in Groups

The real medical revolution of the 1980s was in the accounting department, not in the lab or the operating room. I was reminded of this recently when a national survey showed that a high percentage of doctors feel under pressure to get Medicare patients out of the hospital faster.

Now, most of us want to leave the hospital—a noisy, uncomfortable, dehumanizing place—just as fast as we can. But not at the expense of getting well. And this seems to be one problem with the government's new way of paying for Medicare patients: the danger of sending some people home half-sick. (Lest you think the only people with a problem are your grandparents on Medicare, you should know that your own health-insurance plan is likely to be considering, or has already adopted, some similar system.)

Describing the subtleties of the new system would take a whole book, but here is a short look at how it works, and at some of the questions it raises:

The government has set up some 470 categories of illness or injury that might bring you to a hospital: a broken leg, for example, or pain in the chest. (If you don't fit into one of these diagnosis-related groups, or DRGs, you're likely to end up in a medical textbook as something brand-new.) For each DRG, the feds have calculated the average hospital cost in each region, and set a standard amount they will pay a hospital for complete treatment of that condition. If your stay is longer than the average, the hospital still gets only the standard amount, and will lose money on the extra days. If your stay is shorter than the set amount, the hospital still gets the full amount, and makes an extra profit on you.

A hospital, facing increased competition and a tight economy, has to figure every penny. Many administrators say the DRG amount often isn't enough, and their survival is threatened. Because of these complaints, the government has made the rules a little more flexible and refigures some payments periodically.

Meanwhile, there are other steps a hospital could take to deal with the DRG pinch—steps that are ethically questionable. It could screen Medicare patients more rigorously, taking only those least likely to have complications and sending the others to county hospitals. It could be more aggressive about transfer, shipping out a patient as soon as there were signs it would be a longer-than-average stay. Since "no code" orders—not to resuscitate elderly and terminally ill patients—are becoming more common, and since the criteria are often ambiguous, a hospital could encourage such orders, not out of mercy but as a way to shorten the average stay. A hospital that found it was consistently losing money on DRG payments to its "preemie" unit could close the unit—or raise the birth-weight at which it would attempt resuscitation.

The DRG system worries doctors too. They're concerned because they are the ones who decide when a patient can go home. They're afraid hospitals will lean on them to discharge patients earlier—and, indeed, 48 percent in that recent AMA survey said they already feel "unduly pressured" to do so.

Most hospitals now have computer programs that can list the medical staff according to the average length of stay of each doctor's Medicare patients. If Dr. Bones' patients in DRG 122, "acute myocardial infarction without complications, discharged alive," stay on the average three days longer than those of other doctors, the administration at Angel of Mercy General is going to be interested. At the least, they'll want to ask the doctor why he or she is so far from the average; why, in statistical terms, he's an *outlier*. At the worst, they'll hint that her or his privileges are in danger—unless the lengths of stay begin to come closer to the norm.

The temptation is strong for a doctor to give in to such pressure. Or to escalate his or her diagnosis, moving the patient into a group with a longer allowable stay—a practice already labeled *DRG creep*. The physician is thus caught in the middle: being forced for the patient's sake to be on one hand a liar, or on the other hand, an outlier.

We're Already Rationing Health Care

Mention "rationing of health care" and you can count on one overwhelming response: anger. The response is usually personal and emphatic: "You're not keeping my dad from getting a heart transplant!"

But we're already rationing health care. Even if more of the national budget were going into health care instead of military hardware, for example, there isn't enough money to do everything we know how to do in medicine. So, like the parent who says, ''You can have the bike or the train set for Christmas, but not both,'' we set limits and require choices.

Unfortunately, the way we make these choices in health care is erratic and often unjust. Consider the basis for many decisions:

• **Big employers drawing the line.** *Business Week* says health benefits for auto workers can add $700 to a car's cost. ''Companies increasingly see the elimination of unneeded services as a key to reducing their medical bills.''

• **Emotional appeal.** Of some 4,000 children who need $100,000 liver transplants each year, which ones get them? The ones whose mothers can speak well on television, or win the interest of a newspaper reporter. We ration many of the others out.

• **Geography.** A doctor's freedom to practice where he or she wants has a down side: For some, the doctor is out of reach. There are 100 psychiatrists in one square block on Fifth Avenue, and many whole counties in the United States with no doctor at all.

• **Time.** Getting a doctor's appointment used to take hours; now it can take days, and in a few places, weeks. This rations out many who just can't wait around, dare not be away from jobs, or can't afford child care.

• **Red tape.** Hundreds of children with AIDS were denied life-extending AZT until recently. The ironic reason: a rule, designed to protect kids, that a drug must be tested extensively with adults first.

• **Race and class.** Dr. James Mason, assistant secretary of the United States Department of Health and Human Services explains, ''In this country, we find a pronounced and stubborn disparity between the health status of minority Americans and the rest of us.'' We could correct this; not to do so is a decision about priorities.

• **Inadequate health insurance.** In San Francisco a baby whose parents have no health insurance is 30 percent more likely to get seriously ill or die than one whose parents are insured. And between 1982 and 1986, the proportion of uninsured newborn babies rose 45 percent.

• **Romance with technology.** The decision to fund esoteric technology to save hundreds of lives, at the expense of less exciting preventive measures that might save hundreds of thousands, is a rationing choice. An example is the recent decision by Congress and the National Institutes of Health to spend $3 billion and fifteen years mapping all the human genes.

• **Expensive medicine.** Burroughs Wellcome made AZT—the only drug approved to date to treat AIDS—too expensive for many HIV-infected people. It rationed them right out of the system.

Doctors' fees have risen at a rate roughly double the rise in cost-of-living every year in the last decade. It's no wonder the Washington hearings on plastic surgery were conducted not by Health and Human Services, but by the Small Business Administration.

• **Politics and pressure groups.** One analyst says the repeal of Medicare for catastrophic illness will result in the deaths of 4,000 elderly women who can't otherwise afford mammo-grams. Long-term care is severely rationed by repeal of the law, brought on—according to several members of Con-gress—by a vocal and well-organized group of wealthy retired people. The bill was unjust, many feel, in making only the elderly pay for it, but there is little interest now in passing a better one.

You undoubtedly can add to this list. Carry it along, and show the next person who tells you we can't ration health care.

If It Ain't Broke, Don't Bother Me

Yes, we all know that an ounce of prevention is worth a pound of cure. But it's all so boring.

Don't bother me with those dull statistics about cancer being maybe 80 percent preventable, through less pollution and more attention to nutrition. Tell me instead of a $100 million-a-year "war" on cancer, with "magic-bullet" drugs that will zap those bad cells right out of the body and never touch the good ones.

Don't bother me with the dispute over education as a way to conquer AIDS. Let the fundamentalists and the educators fight over whether S-E-X should be mentioned or not. Tell me instead about the space shuttle zooming up into the never-never, with a little piece of the AIDS virus aboard in a sealed tube, part of a fascinating experiment. Maybe they'll develop drugs to fight the disease, NASA says.

Forget then-Surgeon General Koop, who said the amount of fat in your diet "can influence your long-term health prospects more than any other action you might take," except for heavy smoking or drinking.

Forget the research proving that jobs with high psychological demands, plus little control for the worker, triple the risk of heart attack among men.

Tell me instead of transplants, electric hearts, miracle drugs, and bypass surgery to fix the damage afterward.

Tell me of the dramatic war on drugs, not of the revelation that the Pentagon encouraged military pilots to use uppers to stay alert on a long flight and downers to sleep afterward.

Ignore the news story about the 7 million latchkey children in

144

the United States, and the fact that there are daycare facilities for only 30 percent of the children who need them.

If we have to talk about raising children, read me instead the news story about the fifty-five children from the "Nobel sperm bank" in Escondido, where they have the very best genes and the most sophisticated technology.

No, don't remind me of the mother, scientifically selected from among scores of applicants and impregnated with a Nobel prize-winner's sperm, who turned out to have had two previous children taken away from her for their own protection.

High-tech, that's the name of the game. Cures. Therapy. Procedures. The excitement is in seeing mortally sick people become well, in seeing the crippled walk. Prevention is snoozeville; if it ain't broke . . . don't bother me.

I see that U.S. District Court Judge Stanley Sporkin was out of step. He ruled that the government had illegally blocked Medicare payments for home visits to hundreds, maybe thousands of elderly and disabled people.

The judge wrote: "Because [the government is] unwilling to provide part-time daily home health services, many people needlessly have been forced to make the cruel choice between forgoing needed care or submitting to institutionalization in a nursing home or hospital."

Forget that home care is less costly in the long run, that it can prevent some conditions from becoming acute—and really expensive. Remember that the short-term profit is not in visiting nurses, but in filling nursing homes and hospital rooms.

Surgery to close bedsores is something we can budget for. It challenges the best in medicine. Having a nurse's aide drop by to turn the patient, so bedsores won't develop in the first place, is not nearly as interesting. It doesn't keep the wheels of medical commerce spinning, either.

You can't blame the politicians. They're giving us what we want. Sanitation is boring. Good nutrition is a drag. Education is a vague and dull subject. Warnings on cigarette packs are a violation of our civil rights.

And using three-tenths of 1 percent of all our health care money for health promotion and disease prevention? Yeah, that's about right.

Found! A Cure for Death!

The one belief we all seem to share is that we're not going to die.

Ninety-five percent of us believe that the *Reader's Digest* will be out next month—or at least the month after—with a paper flap on the front that says: "FOUND! A Cure for Death!" The miracle of modern medicine, we're convinced, will push death farther and farther away, until at last it's no longer a threat.

I'm not talking about life after we leave this earth. I mean the widespread belief that not only is life expectancy on the rise, but that it will go on rising indefinitely. Well, you may be interested in the latest figures—reliable research on just how many of us will die, at least as far as this mortal coil is concerned. The figure is 100 percent.

Unfortunately, the results of our refusal to believe this figure are more serious than those from other widespread delusions— that Elvis is alive, for example.

In an important book, *Setting Limits: Medical Goals in an Aging Society,* bioethics pioneer Daniel Callahan argued that it may be this search for perfect health and for indefinitely extended years that has caused today's health care crisis. It's not just the mechanics of health care, or the techniques of financing it, Callahan believes. It's our goals, our "deeper premises," that have brought us so close to disaster. "We have come to . . . desire what we cannot any longer have in unlimited measure—healthier, extended life. The projections (of future health care costs) tell me that we are going to have to change, and change not just the mechanics of our system, but our way of thinking about and understanding illness, life, health, and death."

Any thoughtful observer can see that our pursuit of perfect health and the resultant immortality have led us to spend more and more on high-tech treatment for fewer and fewer people. The miracle of science is lived out daily in intensive-care units and in kidney dialysis centers. We laud it in the cool skill of the transplant surgeon, the computer that locates the needed organ, and the chartered jet that rushes it cross-country. We'll interrupt the news to find a liver for a little girl whose own has failed. We'll give all-out treatment at $1,500 a day to give a few more weeks of life to a man in an irreversible coma. We intend to do everything we know how, for everybody who needs it.

The idea of setting limits rarely comes up. When it does—as when a county in California tried setting realistic priorities for its health care budget—public outrage drowns out the message.

The impossible dream is not a new one. In 1795, the Marquis de Condorcet, philosopher and mathematician, suggested "that this perfection of the human species might be capable of indefinite progress; that the day will come when death will be due only to extraordinary accidents or to the decay of the vital forces, and that ultimately, the average span between birth and decay will have no assignable value."

The result of such beliefs is clear. Health costs are increasing twice as fast as the cost of living, and are expected to triple, to $1.5 trillion a year, in the next decade.

Eventually, Callahan says, we will be forced to admit that our goals are not only unreachable, but harmful overall.

> We must persuade people—those people who are ourselves—
> that we will have to endure illness and death, convince ourselves
> that we are wrong in thinking we no longer have to endure
> disease. . . . We will have to be persuaded that our desire for
> progress, understandable enough, can be preserved but now
> pointed in a different direction, one designed to enrich and
> intensify, not to enlarge and conquer.''

Universal Access to Health: Can It Fly?

Whenever somebody starts telling you that we can't afford a better health care system, think about Huffman's prairie. It is a broad, shallow valley east of Dayton, Ohio, where in 1904 an aeroplane could be seen in action—rising as high as 100 feet in the air, venturing out for as long as five minutes in a broad circle and returning to the takeoff point. The Wright brothers were back from a winter in Kitty Hawk, N.C., and were improving their aeroplane and their flying skills.

You could watch, if you were one of the thousands who rode the interurban train along the edge of the valley every day between Dayton and the towns east. But few of the passengers mentioned the sight. Nor did the Dayton papers ever send a reporter. The reason was simple: Nobody believed it could be done. No matter what their eyes tried to tell them, they knew a flying machine was impossible.

Well, look out the window, folks. The same thing has been

going on for years in arguments about health care. Most of us know that a comprehensive system—fair, efficient, and covering every person—would be impossibly expensive. We "know" this, and we are wrong.

With enthusiastic nudges from those who profit most in the health care industry, we've bamboozled ourselves. While friends and neighbors around us sicken and die for lack of decent care, we've resolutely ignored the alternatives. To see how strong this self-deception is, look at the evidence in any one of dozens of countries—every industrialized nation, in fact, but us and South Africa.

Consider Canada's system, described in an address in Berkeley, California, by Professor Evelyn Shapiro of the University of Manitoba.

Canada spends less on health care than we do. Less per person each year, and less (in percent) of its Gross National Product.

But it has national health insurance, administered by the provinces. Under this plan:

• Since 1971, every Canadian has had insurance that covers all hospital and doctor expenses. (In some provinces, this has been going on since 1952.)

• Most provinces also cover full cost of living in a nursing home.

• People can choose their own doctors, who continue among the top 1 percent of all income earners.

• The system has overwhelming support from the public; it is backed by the major political parties and the health care professions.

• The level of care hasn't suffered; Canada ranks ahead of the United States in such indexes as infant mortality, heart attack survival, and cancer survival.

Briefly, here's how it works: After each visit, your doctor

submits a claim card to the proper provincial agency and is paid according to a fee schedule negotiated between the medical association and the government. If a hospital stay is necessary, the cost is covered under an annual budget negotiated with each institution; a local board of directors runs the hospital. A nurse and a social worker will assess whether you need help at home in order to leave the hospital. Occupational therapy, physical therapy, attendants, or nurses are covered for as long as you need them. The money comes mostly from provincial and federal budgets; some is from low premiums paid on a sliding scale.

"It's a wonderful feeling," a Canadian friend, a retired teacher, told me. "One just doesn't have the terrible worry about how to pay if one gets sick." The bottom line is that all Canadians have access to decent health care, yet with much less drain on the economy.

How can this be? How do they get more for less?

A major point, Professor Shapiro says, is that administration by the provinces cuts out a whole extra layer of paper-shuffling by private and semi-public insurance plans. The incentive is to minimize cost, not maximize profit. Cost control is tough and effective.

By contrast, more than 20 percent of what we spend on health, from aspirin to artificial hearts, goes to administration—about $100 billion a year. It costs us $1.76 for the various public and private entities to process a Medicare claim; in Saskatchewan, the comparable cost is 14 cents.

The beauty of Canada's plan is the bottom line:

For 12 percent of our GNP, we're getting a patchwork program that leaves 37 million people uncovered and places us 14th among the nations in infant mortality. Canada spends 9 percent.

Can Our Health Care System Get Well?

Is it possible that at last, at long last, we are going to make a certain minimum of health care available to every American? Don't bet on it yet. But after seventy-five years, the odds are changing.

In one of the few worthy moments of the 1988 presidential campaign, Jesse Jackson confronted us, not with the usual statistics, but in Baptist pulpit language, outraged at "a hospital admitting room where somebody tonight is dying because they cannot afford to go upstairs—to a bed that's empty, waiting for someone with insurance to get sick."

Jackson wasn't the first to discover that something is wrong with the way we take care of—or fail to take care of—sick people in this country. But he had the national opportunity and the guts and the ability to sum up an explosion of concern. Nationwide polls show that more than 70 percent of the people want some form of universal health care. In fabled conservative Orange County, California, the figure is 75 percent.

We're wising up. Suddenly there's a wider awareness that, under our patchwork, cottage-industry, fee-for-service, stock-holders-first system, we spend a bigger part of our money for health care than any other country in the world.

At the same time:

• Studies document a steady rise in cholesterol, blood pressure, and blood sugar levels among older patients—the result of cutting Medicare and closing clinics.

• The people of fourteen other nations have a longer life expectancy; twenty-six nations have better heart-attack recovery and eighteen nations have fewer babies die in their first year.

• Doctors, who should be advocates for the patient, face increasing pressure to shorten hospital stays. Hospitals, fighting for their lives in the money crunch, use computers to identify

151

those doctors whose patients tend to cost more than the government will pay.

• People with AIDS whose health insurance went down the drain when they lost their jobs find it costs $175 a week or more for a drug that might extend their lives—a drug developed at federal expense, but now making profits for its British manufacturers as one of the most expensive medicines on the market.

• A man dies en route from one hospital to the other because the state has drastically cut its contribution to the counties for health care for the poor, and the institutions that can provide free care are dwindling.

• A nine-year-old cries as the emergency-room doctor cuts a fishhook from his hand; it isn't the physical pain, but knowing that his mother doesn't know where the money is coming from to pay the doctor.

General awareness of such problems, and the willingness to be realistic about the reasons, are signs of hope. Another is equally pragmatic: Big business is worried about employee health costs, which grow 20 percent a year.

They're aware that Canada, with a unified, efficient plan, covers everybody for less of their GNP than we do. They see Sweden, with a higher percentage of older people than we have, spending 15 percent less of its GNP and getting universal coverage. They see in New Zealand a universal health system that has worked for fifty years.

In the United States, they see a hodge-podge system; the only thing that exceeds the paperwork is the profit each institution and entrepreneur siphons off.

When General Motors and Exxon start demanding change, change is more likely.

And a final reason: Maybe we really are beginning to

remember what kind of a people we are. Maybe we're finally abandoning that shibboleth of shriveled souls, that mean and indefensible idea: "The poor are less deserving than the rest of us." It's no longer fashionable to say it out loud, but this ghastly distortion of the scriptures is still the philosophy behind most opposition to universal health care. We're beginning to realize that fairness, decency and caring have been in partial eclipse, shadowed by the bogey-man rhetoric about "socialized medicine." We're realizing the real question is this: Is health care a saleable luxury, like tanning parlors, Caribbean cruises, and cars that will do 120 miles an hour?

Or is it an essential of a humane community, like roads and public schools—a service that we all band together to pay for because we owe it to one another? Try saying "socialized education." "Socialized police." "Socialized firefighting." And listen to Jesse Jackson's question from the speech mentioned earlier: "The poor work in hospitals. They wipe the bodies of those who are sick with fever and pain. . . . And yet when they get sick, they cannot lie in the bed they made up every day." Was Jackson right? "America, that is not right. We are a better nation than that. We are a better nation than that."

Meanwhile, All Around Us . . . An Afterword

My brother Dave and I were eating lunch in his tin-roofed house in the Nigerian bush, looking out at the sun-browned patchy grass and gnarled trees, when he said, "There comes the bush ambulance."

He pointed in the distance, to six men, shouldering a crude stretcher with a cloth-wrapped body on it. Before I could ask what was going on, Dave was loping down the hill toward the hospital. But an hour and a half later he was back, in the loose shirt and pants of a surgeon.

"She had been in labor for three days," he said. "Her pelvis was too small to deliver normally. We did a Cesarean, and they're both OK. It took them twelve hours to get her here. But if they hadn't brought her in, she'd have died."

Out of nowhere, I had a lump in my throat. "It must be a great feeling, to save a life like that—somebody who certainly would have died. . . ."

"Frustrating is more like it," he said. "If she'd had a decent diet when she was growing up, she probably wouldn't have had this trouble. And there are so many more like her, who never get brought in."

He talked about the futility. The Hausa, a nomadic people, sleep outdoors, and on cold nights Hausa mothers lay their naked babies near the campfire to sleep. Now and then a baby rolls into the flames; the ones who survive have terrible burns. Dave, a board-certified surgeon in a well-equipped United Methodist mission hospital, often did skin grafts on babies like this.

"But families that have learned to wrap the babies or dress them at night during the cold months don't have to put them next to the fire to keep them warm. The kids don't get burned."

He said one of the most common killers of babies in the Third World is diarrhea. The conditions that cause it usually have a short life, but the dehydration can be fatal. All over the world, there are tropical hospitals with sophisticated intravenous setups to snatch the babies back from death by replenishing the fluids and restoring the electrolyte balance.

"But in the villages that have a local health teacher, mothers learn to mix salt and sugar in boiled water and feed it to the babies a little at a time while they're sick. They don't get dangerously dehydrated. They don't die, and they don't end up in the hospital.

"I'm beginning to realize that health isn't primarily about

medicine. It isn't mostly about doctors and nurses and hospitals.''

That was in 1969, and change was ahead for both of us. I was about to enter the brand-new field of bioethics, and Dave was about to make the drastic change from surgery to public health.

In the two decades since, I've spent my days with the issues in this book: moral issues in modern Western medicine. They're the dilemmas you and I must live with, and they're not trivial. But it would be a mistake to leave the impression that I think this is all there is to sickness and health.

At widely spaced family reunions over the years, Dave and I have talked about this—about the way the miracles of modern medicine have blinded us to what sickness and health are really about. I became increasingly aware of an irony: that the ''less civilized'' Third World had more to teach us about health than we could teach them.

The ideas weren't new. It's just that we in the West had forgotten them. A few examples:

• **Health involves the whole person.** A thousand miles back in the Nigerian bush, and later for nine years as doctor to the Seminoles in the Everglades, Dave learned to appreciate the work of the local healers—the witch doctors and the medicine men and women. He referred patients to them, and they referred patients to him. Like most of the other ''less civilized'' people of the world, they didn't see the body as a separate machine, but as part of a whole that included mind and spirit.

They knew that we are more inclined to get sick when our feelings and our relationships are troubled. We're more likely to be well when we're in loving relationships and our mind, body, and spirit are in harmony. This is just as true in an American city as in a remote Burmese village.

Humankind has known this for thousands of years. It is central to most religions. The idea permeates the Hebrew and Christian scriptures, and is central to the Christian faith. It's no coincidence that *whole, holy,* and *healing* have the same root.

Churches are beginning to give more than lip service to this idea; many in the United States look to the example of a church-run health clinic in Kingston, Jamaica, where members of the sponsoring congregation work alongside the doctors and nurses, where services of prayer and healing are integral in the program, and where a prayer partner from the congregation is assigned to each patient.

• **Good health is a community matter.** A movement called "community-based medicine" is catching on in countries around the world. It's based on the old truth that people, given a chance to express themselves, know more about their own needs than an outsider, no matter how scientifically trained.

People of a neighborhood discuss what they see as their most urgent health problems. When there is agreement on priorities, the community attacks the problem itself or, if appropriate, brings in the proper professionals.

This approach sees patients as more than passive recipients of "care" that is "given"; they are full partners with a valuable contribution to make. And the priorities tend to involve promotion of good health rather than patching up the sick.

• **Health is a justice issue.** "Many broken relationships are cultural or global," Dave has written. "It is generally accepted that poverty, a result of widespread greed, is the major cause of illness in the world."

A friend told me of meeting a woman in Manila whose little boy had died that day of bronchitis. My friend's young daughter, visiting the Philippines with them, had bronchitis the same day.

"But she was in good health; with good medical care and some antibiotics, she recovered in a few days."

But the woman and her son, poor and ill-nourished, had just fled their burning village in an area devastated by civil war. Medicine had not been enough to cure the son of the real killer diseases: poverty, oppression, alienation, and fear.

■ ■ ■

So it's more complicated than it looks at first. Wrestling with health issues means more than struggling with the dilemmas raised by the technology of modern medicine, as useful and God-given as that medicine may be.

It also means helping to create loving, trusting communities—in our families, neighborhoods, nations, and world.

And it means battling with all our might against injustice, wherever in the world it is causing sickness and death.

BIBLIOGRAPHY
IF YOU WANT TO KNOW MORE . . .

*D*espite the mystique of the "expert," nearly anyone can handle the moral decisions modern medicine demands. It doesn't take a graduate degree—just a little common sense, some information (almost none of it technical), and some careful thought about your beliefs and values.

Here are some helpful sources if you'd like to know more.

Beauchamp, Tom L., and James F. Childress. *Principles of Biomedical Ethics.* New York: Oxford University Press, 1979.

Barbour, Ian. *Science and Secularity: The Ethics of Technology.* New York: Harper & Row, 1970.

Bayer, Ronald. *Private Acts, Social Consequences: AIDS and the Politics of Public Health.* New York: Free Press, 1989.

Callahan, Daniel. *What Kind of Life? The Limits of Medical Progress.* New York: Simon & Schuster, 1990. Is there a humane and just way to balance rising costs and limited resources?

Chesler, Phyllis. *Sacred Bond.* New York: Vintage, 1989. Uses the "Baby M" surrogate mother story to look at bioethics issues.

Dixon, Bernard. *Beyond the Magic Bullet.* New York: Harper & Row, 1978. A doctor's prophetic look at medicine.

Grobstein, Clifford. *Science and the Unborn.* New York: Basic Books, 1988. Reasoned, balanced look by a professor of biology.

Hastings Center. *Hastings Center Report.* Sent every other month to members ($38 a year, 360 Broadway, Hastings-on-Hudson, N.Y. 10706). Good resource for anybody with a long-term interest in bioethics issues.

Humphrey, Derek, and Ann Wickett. *The Right to Die.* New York: Harper & Row, 1986. Valuable for its historical and legal background.

Larue, Gerald A. *Euthanasia and Religion: A Survey of the Attitudes of World Religions Toward the Right to Die.* Los Angeles: The Hemlock Society, 1985.

Macklin, Ruth. *Mortal Choices: Bioethics in Today's World.* New York: Pantheon, 1989.

Marty, Martin E., and Kenneth Vaux, eds. *Health/Medicine and the Faith Tradition: An Inquiry into Religion and Medicine.* Minneapolis: Fortress Press, 1983.

Medwar, P. B. *The Threat and the Glory*. New York: HarperCollins, 1990. Challenging essays by the late Nobel scientist/philosopher.

Pelletier, Kenneth R. *Mind as Healer, Mind as Slayer*. New York: Dell, 1977. A landmark in wholistic medicine.

Ramsey, Paul. *The Patient as Person*. New Haven and London: Yale University Press, 1970. Written by a United Methodist who taught ethics at Princeton. He left work that still challenges.

Robertson, John A. *The Rights of the Critically Ill*. New York: Bantam. One of a valuable series of paperbacks by various publishers, updated regularly, sponsored by the American Civil Liberties Union. Other titles include *The Rights of Doctors and Nurses and Allied Health Professionals, The Rights of Hospital Patients, The Rights of Mental Patients, The Rights of Older Persons, The Rights of Physically Handicapped People,* and *The Rights of Mentally Retarded Persons.*

Sabatier, Renee. *Blaming Others: Prejudice, Race and Worldwide AIDS*. Philadelphia: New Society, 1989. Produced by the Norwegian Red Cross and the Panos Institute.

Schramm, Carl J., ed. *Health Care and Its Costs: Can the U.S. Afford Adequate Health Care?* New York: W. W. Norton, 1987.

Stevens, Rosemary. *In Sickness and in Wealth*. New York: Basic Books, 1989. How the hospital idea went astray.

Winslade, William J., and Judith Wilson Ross. *Choosing Life or Death: A Guide for Patients, Families and Professionals*. New York: Free Press, 1986.

Yamamoto, Keith, and Charles Piller. *Gene Wars: Military Control over the New Genetic Technologies*. New York: William Morrow, 1990. Dr. Yamamoto is vice-chair of the Department of Biochemistry and Biophysics at the University of California-San Francisco.